INITIS

CONGESTION OF THE CONNECTIVE TISSUES

by

ANDREA RABAGLIATI

M.A, M.D, F.R.C.S. (Ed)

Pioneers of Manual Therapy
Volume II

MWI Publishing

Published in Great Britain 2012

by
MASTERWORKS INTERNATIONAL
27 Old Gloucester Street
London
WC1N 3XX
UK

Email: admin@mwipublishing.com
Web: http://www.mwipublishing.com

ISBN: 978-0-9565803-4-4

Book cover by www.mywizarddesign.com

CONTENTS

Foreward to the new edition..9

I. INTRODUCTORY. ON THE TITLE OF THIS BOOK. THE MEANING OF
THE TERM INITIS...12

II. ON THE STRUCTURE AND ARRANGEMENT OF THE CONNECTIVE
TISSUES IN THE BODY; THEIR NAKED EYE AND MICROSCOPIC
ANATOMY. 16

    1. AREOLAR TISSUE..17

    2. FIBROUS TISSUE. 19

    3. ELASTIC TISSUE. 19

III. MICROSCOPICAL STRUCTURE OF CONNECTIVE TISSUE. 20

    development of the connective tissues and blood
    and lymph vessels..20

    The connective tissue is like the ether in the universe 22

    Attraction and repulsion: different views 22

IV. ILLUSTRATIONS SHOWING THE MICROSCOPIC ANATOMY OF THE
CONNECTIVE TISSUES. 25

    Response and appreciation of response: consciousness 27

    The sympathetic system of nerves 30

    Ganglia 31

    Unconscious, visceral, and conscious government..............31

    Nerve-fibres medullated and non-medullated:
    really vaginated and non-vaginated 32

    The sympathetic nervous system an offset from the
    cerebro-spinal system 35

    Contraries as an contradictories...35

V. PHYSIOLOGY OF THE CONNECTIVE TISSUES................................41

    The place of pain not directly perceived 42

VI. THE FUNCTIONAL ACTION OF PARTS IS FELT RATHER THROUGH AFFECTION OF THE COVERINGS OF THE PARTS THAN THROUGH THE INTIMATE STRUCTURE OF THE PARTS THEMSELVES. 43

Neuritis and peri-neuritis: mysitis and perimystis; osteitis and periostitis..43

VII. RHEUMATISM. 45

Meaning of the word rheumatism..45

Rheumatism is congestion or inflammation of the connective tissues..45

Irregularity of symptoms in rheumatism: exaggeration of symptoms in rheumatism 47

VIII. THE URIC ACID THEORY OF RHEUMATISM................................48

Waste-matters in the blood or tissues 48

IX. DIAGNOSIS..49

Value of clinical evidence 49

What iniits may portend..53

X. FURTHER CONSIDERATIONS REGARDING THE FUNCTIONS OF THE CONNECTIVE TISSUES. 54

The connective tissue as the organ of common sensibility and perhaps the feeling of heat and cold, and resistance 54

Effects of a common cause; and cause and effect 55

The whole universe alive 57

Nutritional and political analogies.......................................58

XI. FUNCTIONS OF CONNECTIVE-TISSUE CELLS AND OF NERVE-CELLS. A GENERAL VIEW OF THE RELATIONS OF FUNCTION TO STRUCTURE. 59

XII PELIOSIS 61

Inequality of resistance 61

XIII. ARE DIFFERENCES IN RESISTING POWER TO BE ASCRIBED TO HEREDITY ?..62

What power gifted ancestry with qualities?...........................62

XIV. IS MATTER ETERNAL IN DURATION OR EXTENT? 64

    Matter is constantly vanishing 65

    The eternity of energy real..65

    Simultaneous appearance of animal races at all ages 67

    Variation and mutation...67

XV. INSTANCES OF SIMULTANEOUS SUCCESSION OR OF THE
SIMULTANEOUS APPEARANCE OF WHAT USUALLY OCCUR AS
SUCCESSIVE PHENOMENA IN NATURE. 68

    causation and simultaneous appearance; and
    causation and successive appearance 69

    peliosis 70

XVI. FORMATION OF WEALS ON THE SKIN. 72

XVII. IS THE CONNECTIVE TISSUE THE ORGAN THROUGH WHICH WE
FEEL HEAT AND COLD ? 73

    Heat a quality of kinetic energy 73

XVIII. THE RELATIONS BETWEEN THE CONNECTIVE TISSUE AND THE
LYMPH. 75

    No lymphatic system in invertebrata 75

    The lymphatic system open into the blood-vessels.................76

    Various names for initis 77

XIX. SEQUENCES ON INITIS. 78

    dyspepsia or Mal-assimilation a frequent
    occurrence of iniits and its sequelae.....................................78

    Death in cramp and death in collapse 80

    The cause of a low bodily temperature..................................81

XX. THE FREQUENCY OF THE OCCURRENCE OF CASES OF INITIS...83

    A case of initis 85

    Cause of constipation which so often accompanies initis 90

    Opposite causes may induce similar effects...........................90

PART II. SYSTEMATIC AND REPEATED EXERCISES............93

Figures

1. Manipulation of the Shin bone. 95

2 a. and 2b. Manipulation of the Calf of the Leg and also of the Muscles of the Front of the Leg. 103, 104

3. Manipulation of the Foot. 106

4. Pressure movements of the Knee-joint.............110

5 a and b. Self-movements under pressure of the Muscles of the Thighs. 112

6a and b. Self-movements under pressure of the False Joints of the Back (Sacrum) and the muscles of the Buttocks (glutei muscles)...114

The same as 6 a and 6b. 115

7. Manipulation of the bottom of the Spine: tip of Coccyx. 117

8. Manipulation of the Muscles of the Inside of the Thigh: the Adductor Muscles...............................119

9. Manipulation and movement of the Muscles of the Back: The Erector Spinae Muscles. 120

10. Manipulation and pressure movement of the Infra-spinatus Muscle. 125

11. Manipulation and pressure movement of the Trapezius or Shoulder-raising Muscle. 129

12 a and b. Self-movements under pressure of the Muscles of the outside of the Hips; the Tensores Vagina Femoris; also of the Glutei Medii Muscles 131

13 a and b. Self-movements under pressure of the Side Muscles of the lower part of the Body, and of the False Joints of the Back (sacro-illiac-synchondrosis) simultaneously 133

14 a and b. Self-movements under pressure of the front straight Muscles of the Abdomen (Recti Abdominis Muscles) 135

15 a and b. Self-movements under pressure of the Muscles of the back of the Neck and Shoulder (Splenis Colli and Trapezius Muscles) 137

16 a and b. Self-movements under pressure of the Muscles of the front of the Armpits (Pectoralis Major and Minor Muscles)....145

17 a and b. Self-movements under pressure of the Muscles of the back of the Armpit and Shoulder (the Latissimus Dorsi and Infra-spinatus Muscles)..147

18 a and b. Self-movements under pressure of the Muscles of the Joints of the lower Jaw, and of the Masseter Muscles..........148

19. Self massage of the Sterno mastoid Muscle 150

20. Pressure movements to the Sternum or Breast-bone: to prevent attacks of Angina Pectoris....................................151

21. Self manipulation of the Articulation between the Breast-bone and the 5th and 6th left Ribs, in order to prevent attacks of Angina Pectoris..154

22 a and b. Manipulation of the Shoulder and Deltoid Muscles 157

23 a and b. Manipulation of the Triceps Muscle on the back of the Arm 159

24 a and b. Manipulation of the Elbow-joint particularly of the inner side..161

25 a and b. Manipulation of the Extensor Muscles of the Forearm. The Elbow is in Extension 163

26 a and b. Manipulation of the Extensor Muscles of the Fore Arm. The Elbow is in Flexion 164

27 a and b. Manipulation of the wrist Joint..........................165

28. Manipulation of the Muscles between the Thumb and Fore-Finger 167

Foreward

Andrea Rabagliati was born in Edinburgh in 1843 and died in 1930 after a long and distinguished career in medicine. Beginning his career as assistant medical officer in the Bradford Workhouse, England he went on to become a consulting surgeon.

Along with his wife he was instrumental in the setting up of St. Catherine's Home for Cancer and as such became a pioneer in the Hospice movement. Although a distinguished surgeon he was more and more drawn to medical cases, especially in relation to diet. He published numerous books on diet and built up a large consulting practice based on dietetic lines.

The basis of much of his work was the premise that many chronic ailments arose from the excess of food products which led to a stagnation of the lymphatic system. His remedy was a restrictive diet and education in self-help exercises to free the body of restrictions in the connective tissue which he believed brought about all manner of painful conditions.

Although the role of diet and exercise in relation to ill health is now well known, Rabagliati was a true pioneer. This faithful reproduction of his book INITIS shows just how ahead of his time he was. The topics that he addresses will be of great interest to allopathic doctors and natural health practitioners alike.

For more information on Andrea Rabagliati visit www.pranotherapy.com

INITIS

Nutrition and Exercises

Congestion of the Connective Tissues. On some frequently found Symptoms which interfere with the usefulness of Human Life; their seat in the Coverings of Muscles, Nerves and Bones and in the Ligaments and Joints; their Origin in Mal-Nutrition; and their Treatment by Diet, Massage and Self-Movements of the Affected Parts under Pressure.

by

A. RABAGLIATI

M.A, M.D, F.R.C.S. (Ed)

Honorary Consulting Gynaecologist, late Honorary Surgeon Bradford Royal Infirmary; Consulting Surgeon to Bingley Hospital and to the Home for Incurables, Bradford

First published in 1916

I N I T I S.
PART I.
I. INTRODUCTORY. ON THE TITLE OF THIS BOOK. THE MEANING OF THE TERM INITIS.

IN 1905 I wrote a book, chiefly for the purpose of preventing or dissuading women from submitting to mutilating operations for the cure of ailments, real enough, no doubt, but which did not, in my opinion, depend on organic disease of the organs which it was too customary to remove in order to effect a cure. The title of that small book was "On Some Symptoms which simulate Disease of the Pelvic Organs in Women; and their Treatment by Massage and by Self-Movements of Muscles under Pressure." At that time, no doubt, I had in my mind the idea that these symptoms are so common in women as to be more or less peculiar to them, for an alternative title to the book was "On Ovarian Neuralgia." The consequence, or the most important consequence, of the operative treatment of such cases from the patient's point of view was, it was there argued, that the operation did not cure the disease. I do not know whether my efforts have had any effect. I do think that the operation of oophorectomy or removal of the ovaries for pain is a good deal less common than it was; but it might not be just to attribute this good result to my small book. It may be mainly due to a change of fashion. I think, however, that surgeons generally have come to the conclusion that oophorectomy does not cure abdominal pain so often as it was once supposed to do.

My book has been for some years out of print; and on a new edition being required, I have had to consider what form it should take. As I expounded in it the view that the pain complained of was due rather to affection of the muscle-sheaths and nerve-sheaths and of the connective tissues of the body, than to affection of any special organs, so, longer experience has more and more confirmed me in this opinion, for the more patients I see, the more convinced am I that a very large proportion of them are suffering from congestion of the connective tissues. And further, this being so, my attention has been gradually and almost unconsciously directed to the fact that, although the affection is found rather among women than among men, it is by no means exclusively nor even essentially a women's ailment. In so far, indeed, as it is rather a women's ailment than a men's, this is due, not so much to sex differences as to differences of habits as between the sexes. Of course, ovarian neuralgia cannot occur in men, but neuralgia and myalgia and ostealgia can and do; that is, men as well as women may and do suffer from pain and stiffness referred to nerves, muscles and bones.

I quite admit still that women suffer, as a rule, more from these affections than men but still, men suffer from them to a very great extent. And, further than that, the principles and the methods of cure are essentially similar in the two sexes. Even children suffer not infrequently in the same ways. This being so, and as I have come to see the widespread nature of the affection in the body and the frequency of its occurrence in individual cases, it has become necessary to alter the title of the book from one dealing with ovarian or quasi-ovarian neuralgia to one which shall indicate the more general nature of the affection. I have therefore had to consider what title I should choose or in what word I should incorporate the view that the affection is chiefly one of the connective tissues of the body, for (as will shortly appear) the disease is not so much one of nerves, muscles or bones as it is an affection of the envelopes or coverings of these parts. On the whole, I have chosen the term

INITIS

as my new title

The word is connected with the Greek ἴς – Latin- vis or strength—and the intention in choosing the title is to show that the affection is mainly one of the strong or connecting tissues of the body. These are so called because they connect every part of the body with every other. Nor is the word without authority, for in Homer and also in Hippocrates, the term ἰνίον is used of the collection of connective tissue which is found at the nape of the neck, and which serves to connect the head with the trunk. In Latin this is termed the *nucha*. In some animals, as the horse, elephant, etc., this nuchal tissue undergoes extraordinary development, as the life-force introduces it for the purpose of supporting the great weight of the animal's head and allowing it to be held in its place easily, painlessly and efficiently. Properly speaking, the term ought, I think, to have been Syndesmitis (from συνδεσμεῖν, to bind), because the main seat of the affection is in the tissues which bind or connect every part of the body with every other. But the term Syndesmitis has already been appropriated to affections of the ligaments of joints, and it is almost impossible, or at least very difficult, to divert a name from one signification to another, even if the other is a better one.

Affections of the ligaments of joints are no doubt a particular case of what I am calling by the general name Initis. So are affections of tendons, vulgarly called guiders (*tenonitis*, from τένων, a tendon or "guider ") and inquiry into the arrangement of the connective tissues will well repay the labour, since it so closely concerns treatment. Tendons are the cords or bands which are found at the ends of muscles, usually at their insertions, and which serve the purpose of enabling muscles to be attached to bones so as to act as instruments for the movements of bones and of the body in general, that is for motion and locomotion. They are white, glistening and elastic, and differ very much in appearance from the red, fleshy substance of the muscles proper. They are inseparably connected with the sheaths or coverings of the muscles rather than with their red, fleshy tissue; and it is through the functional action of these connective and connecting tissues, rather than by means of the muscle-substance proper, that feelings of aching and fatigue and obscure discomfort are experienced when these tissues are congested. And on the other hand, when these tissues are healthy and free from congestion, we experience feelings of health, lightness, freedom and general well-being.

II. ON THE STRUCTURE AND ARRANGEMENT OF THE CONNECTIVE TISSUES IN THE BODY; THEIR NAKED EYE AND MICROSCOPIC ANATOMY.

Before going on to consider the functions of the connective tissues, or rather, coincidently with doing so, since it is almost impossible to separate structure from what we suppose to be its functions, some attention ought to be given to the anatomy of the parts affected in general Initis. For this purpose, I have drawn freely on Quain's "Elements of Anatomy" for my descriptions, so as to ensure that the clinical observations of the consulting room (for patients suffering from Initis in the ways to be detailed are seldom compelled to be confined to bed) shall be associated with authoritative description of facts of structure. Of course, for the interpretation of the facts (much more important than the facts themselves) every inquirer is himself responsible; and I have no wish to shirk responsibility for my own interpretation.

Interpretation of the facts of organic or organised structure belongs to physiology rather than to anatomy. I have tried to keep the consideration of structure and function, or anatomy and physiology, separate from one another, but it is almost impossible to do so, as the quotations from Quain will show. By the kindness also and courtesy of Messrs Longmans, Green & Co., for which I am very grateful, I have been enabled to reproduce a number of illustrations of the microscopic anatomy of the fibres and cells of the connective tissues of the body. Their study will be as instructive to the general reader as it has been to myself. According, then, to authoritative anatomists, there are three principal elements in connective tissue—viz. "White fibres, elastic fibres and connective tissue corpuscles." The kinds or species of the connective tissues are known as the areolar, the fibrous and the elastic.

1. AREOLAR TISSUE.

"If" (says Quain, 'Elements of Anatomy,' 9th edit., vol. ii., pp. 55-56) "we make a cut through the skin, and proceed to raise it from the subjacent parts, we observe that it is loosely connected to them by a soft filamentous substance of considerable tenacity and elasticity, and having when free from fat, a white, fleecy aspect; this is the substance known as areolar tissue. In like manner the areolar tissue is found underneath the serous and mucous membranes which are spread over various internal surfaces, and serves to attach those membranes to the parts which they invest; and as under the skin it is named 'subcutaneous so in the last-mentioned situations, it is called ' subserous ' and 'submucous' areolar tissue. But on proceeding further, we find this substance lying between the different organs of the body where they are not otherwise insulated, and thence named 'intermediate;' very generally also it becomes more consistent and membranous immediately around these organs, and under the name of the 'investing' areolar tissue affords each of them a special sheath. It thus forms enclosing sheaths for the muscles, the- nerves, the blood vessels and other parts. Whilst the areolar ' tissue might thus be said in some sense both to connect and to insulate entire organs, it also performs the same office in regard to the fine parts of which these organs are made up; for this end it enters between the fibres of the muscles, uniting them into bundles; it connects the several membranous layers of the hollow. viscera, and binds together the lobes and lobules of compound glands; it also accompanies the

17

vessels and nerves within these organs, following their branches nearly to their finest divisions, and affording them support and protection. This portion of the areolar tissue has been named the ' penetrating' ' constituent' or ' parenchymal.' It thus appears that the areolar is one of the most extensively distributed of the tissues. It is, moreover, continuous throughout the body, and from one region it may be traced without interruption into any other, however distant, a fact not without interest in practical medicine, seeing that in this way dropsical waters, air, blood and urine, effused into the areolar tissues, and so in the matter of suppuration when not confined in an abscess, may spread far from the spot where they were first introduced or deposited.

"On stretching out a portion of areolar tissue by drawing gently asunder the parts between which it lies, it presents an appearance to the naked eye of a multitude of fine, soft and somewhat elastic threads, quite transparent and colourless, like spun glass; these are intermixed with fine, transparent fibres, or delicate membranous laminae, and both the ends and laminae cross one another irregularly and in all imaginable directions, leaving open interstices or areolae between them. These meshes are, of course, more apparent when the tissue is thus stretched out; it is plain also that they are not closed cells, as the term ' cellular tissue,' which was formerly used to denote the areolar tissue, might seem to imply, but merely interspaces, which open freely into one another; many of them are occupied by the fat, which, however, does not lie loose in the areolar spaces but is enclosed in its own vesicles. A small quantity of *colourless transparent fluid of the nature of lymph* is also present in the areolar tissue, but, in health *not more than is sufficient to moisten it.*" [Italics mine.—A. R.]

18

2. FIBROUS TISSUE.

"When the fine bundles of connective tissue are disposed for the most part in one or two directions, as in the areolar tissue, they confer a distinctly fibrous aspect to the parts which they compose, accompanied by the acquisition of certain properties, which are mainly due to the parallel disposition of the elements of the tissue, and to the preponderance of the white fibres over the elastic. This *fibrous tissue* is met with in the form of ligaments, connecting the bones together at the joints; it also forms the tendons of muscles, into which their fleshy fibres are inserted, and which serve to attach these fibres to the bones."

These fibrous bands form the coverings of bone (periosteum), also the fibrous covering of the brain (dura mater) and the lining of the skull; the fibrous part of the pericardium or fibro-serous sac in which the heart lies; and also form the coverings of other parts and organs of the body. The fibrous tissue is very strong, but not extensible. It does not, like india-rubber, lengthen and shorten under strain and recoil, or it does so very little indeed.

3. ELASTIC TISSUE.

This tissue is extensible and elastic in the highest degree but is not so strong as ordinary fibrous ligament, and it breaks across the direction of its; fibres when forcibly stretched. It is found in the back of the neck and along the vertebrae of the back joining their arches to one another, and it is also spread over the muscles of the abdomen and assists in the support of the abdominal viscera.

III. MICROSCOPICAL STRUCTURE OF CONNECTIVE TISSUE.

By the courtesy of Messrs Longmans, Green & Co. I am able here to introduce reproductions of figures appearing in the 9th edition of Quain's "Anatomy," vol. ii., pp. 59-62. These figures the reader will do well to study, since nothing probably will be so instructive as they in throwing light on the rationale both of the ways in which these structures may get out of order, and do get out of order in the body, and also as to the proper use of exercises accompanied by proper nutrition or feeding, so as to restore them to health. For the connective tissue, following the branches of vessels and nerves nearly to their finest divisions, cannot be congested without congesting also the coats of the blood and lymph vessels; and still less can it be injured or sprained or ruptured without injuring or tearing these other structures also; and as, of course, the blood vessels and lymph vessels are essentially organs of nutrition, the connective tissues are thus seen to have intimate relations with nutrition also. Thus we read again in Quain (9th edition, vol. ii., p. 198): "Within the body of the embryo, vessels are formed in like manner from cells belonging to the connective tissue." This is, like some statements that are to follow, a fact of development. And we may take it that when in the process of development one structure is developed from another, these two structures are related in function or purpose or use. If the lungs are developed from the digestive tract, as they are, we may take it that the lungs are complementary digestive organs, a conclusion which is of the utmost practical use to us in the treatment and even more in the prevention of respiratory affections such as bronchitis, asthma, pneumonia and consumption. And so with the development of the connective tissues and blood and lymph vessels. If these last are formed from connective tissue cells, it must be

20

because both vessels and connective tissues are intimately related to nutrition. From the description indeed we infer that blood, blood vessels, lymph vessels and connective tissues all arise at once and simultaneously in development. As to the lymph, it exists in the body to twice or thrice the amount reached by the blood.

Whether the presence of so large a quantity of lymph in the body is healthy or unhealthy is a matter for inquiry. The text-book says in the passage quoted that in health the lymph exists in the connective tissue to an extent "not more than is sufficient to moisten it." Whether this statement is compatible with the other made by physiologists that there is twice or thrice as much lymph in the body as there is of blood is a matter for inquiry and consideration. If it should turn out that by the mismanagement of our digestive and nutritional apparatus, the great majority of us have managed to get our bodies into an unhealthy and pathological condition instead of a healthy and physiological one, it would be a strange thing—but it is not impossible. And indeed there are a good many reasons for thinking this likely. At any rate the strange fact remains that very little is said by writers on medicine about the circulation of the lymph in the body, although it is admitted that the volume of it is so much greater than that of the blood. On a proper summing up of the evidence it may turn out that to see the significance of the circulation of the lymph is even more important than to discover the circulation of the blood and to understand its meaning. No doubt the two circulations, that of the blood on the one hand and of the lymph on the other, must be studied together, for they arise together. Thus we find Quain saying ("Anatomy," ninth edition, vol. ii., p. 34) that lymph corpuscles "may also be formed by proliferation of connective-tissue corpuscles." And again (vol. ii., p. 877), "like the blood-vessels, the lymphatic vessels are intimately associated with the connective tissue, and they take their origin in a somewhat similar manner in spaces which are formed in the primitive blastema." (See Fig. 7, representing the jelly of Wharton.)

These quotations from a recognised anatomical authority are the proof of the importance of the relations that exist between the connective tissue and the nutritional organs of the body, and also the proof of the statement that the connective tissue is the most important gland in the body, since it may be said to secrete the lymph and to form its vessels. Rather, I take it, ought we to say that the force of animal life procreates lymph and blood and their vessels, but that it does so in the substance of the connective tissue, which it simultaneously procreates for that purpose. The connective tissue, in short, is like the all-pervading ether in the physical universe, and perhaps also resembles the bonds of good will which ought to unite in harmonious action all kinds of human life. It performs a similar unifying function in the bodily organism which the ether does in the body of the material universe, and which the bonds of good will perform in the sphere of the responsive, intellectual, emotional and spiritual forces usually termed life. Just as the force of gravitation or hylo-dynamic seems to procreate the ether as the vehicle or means by which it may convey itself throughout the infinite space subject to its authority, so zoo-dynamic or the force of animal life seems to introduce or procreate the connective tissue as the vehicle or means by which the whole body (and every organised body) shall be subject to the authority of the life-force. And if we realise that gravitation is a force which attracts or draws together the matter which yields a willing or at least a neutral or passive obedience to its sway, and that apparent repulsion is always the manifestation of a degree of attraction by their surroundings greater than that which exists between bodies apparently repelled from one another, we may perhaps have some further insight into the parallel between the functions of the connective tissue and the ether and also between it and attraction physical, moral and spiritual. Two pith balls similarly electrified fly violently apart from one another, and the balloon filled with hydrogen gas may be said to be repelled from the earth. But if it be true that the pith balls are more attracted to their surroundings than they are to one another, and that because an equal volume of atmospheric air is more attracted to the earth than a similar mass of hydrogen gas, though carrying a car and passengers with it—if this be so, then perhaps apparent repulsion is only a minor degree of attraction, and perhaps there is no repulsion at all. If this could be shown to be true of moral and spiritual things also, it might at first sight seem remarkable. Perhaps, however, it is true that even hate and enmity are only perversions of love, being the proof that we love ourselves so much that we do not hesitate to damage or even destroy our neighbours in order to aggrandise ourselves. The infinite, omnipotent and eternal, energy of which the universe is the manifestation, is one, and all the so-called forces; which it is convenient for us to divide it into, in order that we may comprehend it a little better,are only particular forms or varieties of the one universal energy. When so viewed, hylo-dynamic and zoo-dynamic are found to work alike—as indeed, had we only known it, it was impossible that they should fail to do. The reader who cares to work them out may perhaps find parallels more instructive still.

However, this suggestion of interpretation may be viewed, I set down here another quotation from Quain (vol. ii. p. 201) :

> "It is, however, with the connective tissue of the several textures and organs that the lymphatics are most intimately associated; indeed, as we shall immediately have occasion to notice, these vessels

may be said to take origin in spaces in that tissue. The larger lymphatic trunks usually accompany the deeply-seated blood vessels; they convey the lymph from the plexuses or sinuses of origin towards the thoracic duct."

IV. ILLUSTRATIONS SHOWING THE MICROSCOPIC ANATOMY OF THE CONNECTIVE TISSUES.

The following figures, introduced by the kind permission of Messrs Longmans, Green & Co., the publishers of Quain's "Elements of Anatomy," show the microscopic anatomy of the connective tissues and of some other parts, so that a comparison may be made between them. They are numbered, for the present purpose 1. 2, 3, etc., although numbered 57, 58, 59, 61b in the original form, of which they are copies. The first figure (No. 1 in this series) is a representation of the microscopic anatomy of white fibrous tissue, and shows very well the general arrangement of the filaments of the areolar tissue and

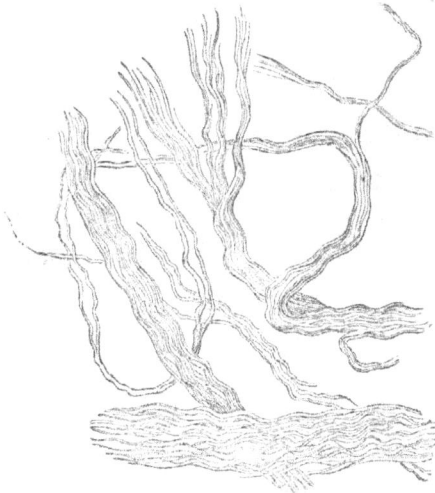

FIG. 1 (Quain, No. 57, vol. ii., p. 59).

its larger and smaller bundles under a magnifying power of 400 diameters. It will require no great stretch of the imagination to see how this structure serves to connect one part of the body with another, and parts of the body with other parts, so as to act as the organ of union and solidarity to the body.

Figure 2 (Quain, No. 58, vol.ii.,v p.60 represents elastic

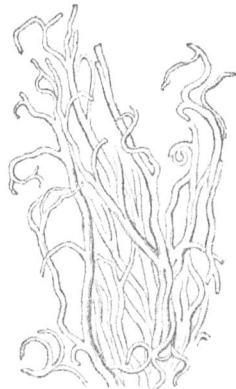

FIG. 2 (Quain, No. 58, vol ii., p. 60).

fibres of connective tissue as found uniting the arches of the vertebrae or jointed bones of the back, magnified about200 diameters.

Figure 3 (Quain, No. 59, vol. ii., p. 60) represents elastic fibres from the ligamentum nuchae of the ox. The figure shows transverse markings on the fibres.

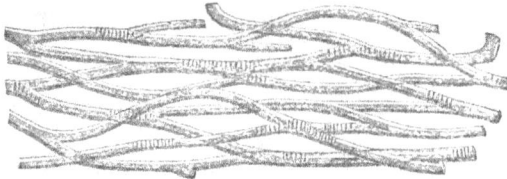

FIG. 3 (Quain, No. 59, vol. ii., p. 60).

Figure 4 (Quain, No. 61b, vol. ii., p. 61) shows the branching of the nearly straight elastic fibres of areolar tissue, and their union into a network of fibres.

It will be noticed that small corpuscular bodies or cocci are seen in this figure. They seem to be lying loose

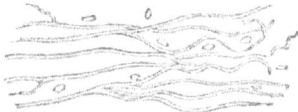

FIG. 4 (Quain, No. 61b, vol. ii., p. 61).

among the fibres of the areolar tissue, and not joined to them by poles as in the next figure. They are probably lymph corpuscles.

In Figure 5 are introduced the cellular elements of the connective tissue. The section is taken from a young guinea-pig and magnified 350 diameters. In the centre of the figure a cell is shown, round, with enclosing wall, cell contents, nucleus and nucleolus, and connected at two sides with filaments which pass into or out of It according to the standpoint from which we view it. On the right hand side of the figure is seen one many branched

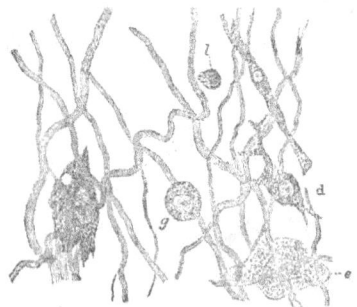

FIG. 5 (Quain, No. 62, vol. ii., p. 62).
Subcutaneous connective tissue of a young guinea-pig; magnified 350 diameters. (d) branched corpuscle; (g) granular corpuscle; (l) leucocyte or migratory cell

or multipolar cell, *d*. It also has its enclosing membrane, its nucleus and nucleolus, and its protoplasmic contents. Just above it is seen a long cell with nucleus, nucleolus and protoplasmic contents; and the cell terminates in a branching or polar end. As we must have a name to denote the function or use or the connective tissue cell, I propose to call it sensible. As the fibre is the apparatus of unity or solidarity, so the cell is the apparatus for the manifestation of sensibility.

There are difficulties in applying words to things, and perhaps still more in applying words to our ideas of things. All tissues are responsive (or apamoebic, from ἀπαμείβομαι I respond) to the life-force that procreates them and inhabits them; but this response is of higher and lower forms, according as higher or lower manifestations of the life force are to be expressed. So we find fibres introduced, for the manifestation or expression of unity, and cells for the manifestation of sensibility. Later figures (Nos. 8 and 9 of this series) will bring into notice a further manifestation of life-force—viz. the *appreciation* of conductivity. The appreciation of unity, and the appreciation of sensibility, but a new set of structures will then be introduced by the life-force for the purpose—viz, nerve-fibres and nerve-cells which are higher in the scale than connective tissue fibres and connective tissue cells. When we study these in the brain and spinal cord, we come into relation with appreciation of conductivity and appreciation, or perhaps recognition, of sensibility and that by using nerve forms the life force introduces apparatus by which it gets to know that it feels, to know that it knows, and even to know that it knows that it knows; or to become fully conscious in the highest sense; if, that is , we ever do rise to conscious knowledge of ourselves, and of our relations to the universe in which we live, and of which we form a small or even infinitesimal and fractional part.

We shall have to consider these points again; so they may be left at this point now with the suggestion to the reader that perhaps the connective-tissue fibres and cells are the apparatus introduced by the life-force for the manifestation of unconscious, or, might one say, not yet conscious, unity, and unconscious or perhaps not yet conscious sensibility; while the cerebro-spinal nerve fibres and the cerebro-spinal nerve-cells are the apparatus for the manifestation of conscious unity and conscious sensibility. If the reader should ask himself or herself how sensibility can possibly be unconscious, that is the very question, or one of them, that I am anxious that he should put to himself. There is even a form of sensibility intermediate between unconscious sensibility and conscious sensibility. This we may term visceral or instinctive sensibility, and on examination we find a third set of structures introduced by the life-force for its manifestation and expression. This is the gangliated or sympathetic system of nerves, as it is called, and a word or two may be said here about it.

Quain ("Elements of Anatomy," 12th edition, vol. i., part 2, p. 307) says :

"The nerves are divided into the cerebro-spinal and the sympathetic nerves. The former are distributed principally to the skin, the organs of the senses, and other parts endowed with manifest sensibility, and the muscles. They are, for the most part, attached in pairs to the cerebro-spinal axis, and, like the parts which they supply, are, with few exceptions, remarkably symmetrical on the two sides of the body. The sympathetic nerves on the other hand, are destined chiefly for the viscera and blood vessels, of which the movements are involuntary, and the natural sensibility is obtuse. They differ also from the cerebro-spinal nerves in having generally a greyish or reddish colour, in their less symmetrical arrangement, and especially in the circumstance that the ganglia connected with them are much more numerous and more widely distributed. Branches of communication pass from many of the spinal nerves at a short distance from their roots, to join, and in fact, to form, the sympathetic, which is thus seen to be merely an offset from the cerebro-spinal centre, as indeed its mode of development (see 'Embryology') would also appear to show."

Now we have already seen that unconscious response, unconscious conductivity, unconscious sensibility and unconscious unity are manifested through the connective tissue, while the appreciation of response, the appreciation of conductivity, the appreciation of sensibility and the appreciation of unity and solidarity are manifested through the cerebro-spinal system. Connective–tissue impressions are probably unlocalised, and sometimes even quite atopic or unplaced, as we may have an affection without knowing with what part of the organism it is connected; while impressions received through the cerebro-spinal nervous system, if not quite localised, are or may be rather more so than those received either through the connective tissue or the sympathetic system of nerves. The place of an affection, however, is probably reached by a process of inference or judgment or reasoning. The process of reasoning being forgotten, localisation may appear to be a direct impression, just as we think we see distance while we really infer it from the comparative visible size and the comparative dimness or clearness of the visible object. Perhaps we might feel localisation directly and not merely infer it, if the structures of the cerebro-spinal nervous system were to reach a much more complex and subtle arrangement than they have now? But however this may be, we may ask ourselves what is the use of the sympathetic system of nerves and in what respects does it differ from that of the connective tissues on the one hand and from that of the cerebro-spinal system of nerves on the other ?

In order to have clear ideas on this question, or in order to have ideas as clear- as we can get, the following facts should be remembered. The sympathetic system of nerves consists, like the connective tissue, and like the cerebro-spinal system of nerves, of fibres and cells. The cells of all three sets of structures agree in being connected or attached and not free or unattached, as are the blood-cells or the lymph—cells which float in a fluid medium, and are not connected with one another by bands or fibres. It was in connection with connected or attached cells that the attribute of sensibility was used when it was said that cells were interpolated by the force of life for the manifestation of sensibility. Had we been speaking of the functions of free or unattached cells we should hardly have been entitled to speak of them as sensible; and I suppose that the term responsive would have been more suitable. But all tissues are responsive, and indeed terminology is very defective, mainly because it is somewhat difficult to have clear ideas regarding the expression of functions through tissues. There are, indeed, two sets of considerations which must be kept distinct in our minds when studying this subject. There are what may be called the properties of tissues which are related to the constitution of the structures; and there are their functions which are related to their connections. A cell will always be responsive whatever be its connections. But a cell unattached and floating in a fluid medium will be responsive simply, while a connective-tissue cell united with another by a fibre will manifest sensibility, though still unconscious sensibility. A cell of the sympathetic system of nerves again, united to its neighbours in a ganglion, will manifest what we may term organic or instinctive sensibility; and if the ganglion is connected by strands or bands with the liver, there may be a feeling of affection under stimulation which may be obscurely referred to the right side. In this way instinctive unity may be reached, or perhaps what may be termed organic unity, such as is manifested by ants and bees, who, though they have no brains proper, yet do perform the most wonderful personal and social functions by means of the ganglia they possess.

A ganglion is a collection of cells intimately joined to one another for the purpose of acting together and so of controlling the actions of the parts of the body with which their fibres are connected. It is connected with the Greek word, γαγγαλίζειν, to tickle or excite. Ganglion is therefore quasi ganglion. The sympathetic system of nerves through its unsheathed fibres and through its ganglia controls or is the means adopted by the life-force to control the life of the viscera such as the liver, kidneys, intestines, spleen, blood vessels, etc.; and hence secretion and excretion and nutrition generally, with blushing, pallor, etc., are under its control and government. It is difficult to express these differences of function in words which shall have and maintain always clear and definite meaning; but perhaps we may say that the connective tissue is the organ for unconscious government, that the sympathetic nervous system is the organ for visceral or organic or instinctive government, and that the cerebro-spinal nervous system is the organ for conscious government?

If the reader is not satisfied with these definitions and if he says that they do not seem to be mutually exclusive, well, this must be admitted. But are any of the departments of nature mutually exclusive of one another? And is not the conclusion that all the departments of nature merge into one another by gradations so insensible that you cannot tell where one ends and where the other begins—is not this the reflection which forces itself on the student more frequently than any other ? As if to emphasise the force of this conclusion in the instance before us, we find from Quain, as already mentioned, that "the sympathetic is... merely an offset from the cerebro-spinal centre." Study of its development leads to the same conclusion. Is it any wonder then that it is somewhat difficult to differentiate clearly between the functions of the connective tissues, those of the sympathetic system of nerves, and those of the cerebro-spinal system? Time will no doubt help to elucidate these` difficulties and give us clearer knowledge. At present they must be left as they are. I cannot, at least, make a better attempt at differentiation of function among these three sets of structures, and shall feel grateful to anyone who will offer clearer explanations.

The sympathetic nervous system differs in still another particular from the cerebro-spinal nervous system besides the difference that it is gangliated, or ganglionated, while the cerebro-spinal is not. This is (and it is often by anatomists stated to be the chief difference between the two), that the sympathetic nerve-fibres are mainly without sheaths, while the fibres of the cerebro-spinal nervous system are provided with them as a rule. The distinction is expressed- by saying that the cerebro-spinal fibres are medullated, while the sympathetic fibres, are non-medullated. This is an unfortunate use of words, because the medulla is the centre or inner part, or marrow or kernel of a structure; and both the cerebro-spinal system and the sympathetic system are undoubtedly medullated——that is, they possess a central portion. The distinction ought to have been expressed by saying that the cerebro-spinal fibres are sheathed or vaginated (not medullated) (vagina, a sheath), while the sympathetic fibres (called often fibres of Remak) are unsheathed or unvaginated (not non-medullated). However, I suppose for the present we must continue to understand the medullated nerve-fibre as meaning the sheathed fibre, and the non-medullated nerve fibre as meaning the unsheathed fibre. And we must understand that the cerebro-spinal system of nerves is medullated, while the sympathetic system of nerves is non-medullated. As the connective tissue forms the sheath when there is one, it is difficult to say whether the connective tissues themselves are sheathed or unsheathed; There may be linings or sheaths of sheaths, or coverings of coverings; for anatomists speak of a "medullary sheath; and also of a primitive sheath which is "a delicate membranous tube outside of all, termed the nucleated sheath of Schwann, the primitive sheath, or the neurolemma." And in a note it is said: "The term neurilemma or neurolemma was formerly applied to the connective tissue sheath of the funiculus, which is now known as the perineurium" (Quain, "Anatomy," 9th edition,vol. i., part 2, p. 309).

The presence of a medullary sheath and a primitive sheath may well raise questions as to the precise differences of function subserved by these two structures—questions, however, which it is easier to ask than to answer. The force of life, however, is very subtle, and the procreations which it introduces, to serve as the means of expressing its finely differentiated requirements or unconscious intentions, are as subtle as itself. The reader will perhaps ask himself questions as to guidance and direction by the conscious of the unconscious in the procreations of structure—questions which I join him in pondering, if I am unable to solve them. A fact, indeed, not yet considered seems to add to this difficulty, for on the page of Quain last referred to, we find it stated that "there are medullated fibres in which the primitive sheath is absent, and other fibres and prolongations of fibres, in which there is no sheath whatever to the axis-cylinder." It seems also to be the case that the axis-cylinder is the chief anatomical constituent of the nerve-fibre. The axis-cylinder is the essential or central part of every nerve-fibre. In trying to differentiate, then, between the functions of the sympathetic nerves and of the cerebro-spinal system we find as a rule that the former are sheathed while the latter are unsheathed; also that the former are gangliated while the latter are not. But as if to emphasise the difficulty of separating between the properties of the two, we find that occasionally the cerebro-spinal nerves are unsheathed. And nextly, as to the gangliation of the sympathetic nerves and the non-gangliation of the cerebro-spinal, surely the corpora striata and optic thalami may be viewed as ganglia, while anatomists often view the convolutions of the brain as ganglia also. If anatomical differences, while generally preserved, sometimes fail us, it becomes very difficult to separate the properties of the sympathetic nerves from those of the cerebro-spinal; and while I still think that on the whole the functions of the former are instinctive while those of the latter are voluntary or conscious, still it is occasionally almost impossible to separate the instinctive response of the viscera from the voluntary response of the brain or cerebrum. The conclusion seems therefore to be forced on us that the instinctive and the voluntary shade off from one another, or merge into one another by gradations so insensible that we cannot really say where one ends and where the other begins.

A surer means of separating the functions of the sympathetic system of nerves from those of the cerebro-spinal system is to remember that on the whole the former are related or distributed to the viscera, like the stomach, the liver, the kidneys, and the (so-called) involuntary muscles, while the latter are related or distributed to the skin, the so-called voluntary muscles and the sense-organs. These two sets of structures again roughly correspond to the inner and outer parts of the body, so that we may perhaps say that the sympathetic nervous system is for the expression of sensations connected with inside parts, while the cerebro-spinal system is for the expression of sensations connected with outside parts. But when we reflect that the sympathetic system is an "offset,?" to use Quain's word, from the cerebro-spinal system, and when we further reflect that the fibres of the one are distributed in many cases, along with those of the other, we are compelled to conclude that it is almost impossible to separate the functions of the one from those of the other. For my own part, I cannot say that I am surprised at this conclusion, for the same force of life (zoo-dynamic) seems to procreate both, and when one comes to reflect that zoo-dynamic is one of the varieties of the universal energy by which all things do subsist, the necessary relations of the various parts of the universe to one another come perhaps to be a little better understood.

Note.—The reflection that the functions of the involuntary and the voluntary nervous systems merge into one another by gradations so insensible that we can hardly say where one ends and where the other begins is one instance which, the text suggests, is a constantly recurring one to the student of nature. And so it is. Otherwise we may say that the universe is full of contraries, while there are very few contradictories. Contraries differ from one another only in degree, while contradictories are mutually exclusive of each other for ever. Instances of the former are almost innumerable, as e.g. .light and dark, day and night, black and white, long and short, hot and cold, right and wrong, well and ill, physiological and pathological, sane and insane, living and dead, conscious and unconscious, voluntary and involuntary, normal and abnormal, etc., etc. The test of the contrary or of contraries will generally conform to the formula that we can say that A can usually be made to conform to its contrary B by insertion of the words *"rather,"* or *"sometimes"* or *"partly."* Thus it is equally true if we say that a line is rather long or rather short, that a colour is rather dark or rather light; or in weight, that a mass is rather heavy or rather light; or that in morals an action is sometimes right and sometimes wrong, or partly right and partly wrong; or partly physiological or normal and partly pathological or abnormal, etc., etc. In the case of contradictories, however, we cannot adopt these expressions. I know of only one pair of contradictories, though it may be put in different ways. Either, it seems to me, life makes material organisation, or material organisation makes life; either energy makes material substance, or material substance makes energy. And in the end either God makes an infinite eternal omnipotent merciful and just universe, or an infinite eternal omnipotent merciful and just universe makes God. We cannot, or at least I cannot, say, as in the former cases, that it is rather the one and rather the other; that it is sometimes the one and sometimes the other; or that it is partly the one and partly the other. It seems to me that I am compelled by the constitution of my nature to accept one or other of these alternatives, and that I am precluded by the same constitution for ever from the attempt to hold both as true.

At least, however, and whatever answers we may give to these suggestions, we see introduced in this Figure 5, not only cells as at *g*, but cells which are branched or polar, or even multipolar, as at *d*. As these poles, or some of them, pass into the connective-tissue-fibres, it is evident that we have here an apparatus introduced, not only for sensibility but even for consociated, or perhaps we might say for associated, sensibility. This apparatus is even more highly developed in Figure 6. Figure 6 shows connective-tissue corpuscles highly magnified, and shows also a large number of poles or processes which may and often do proceed from them. On examination we find how intricate and complicated is the apparatus introduced by the life-force, with its lamellae or plates (one of which is seen projecting its edge to the observer), its fibres and its cells, non-polar, bi-polar and multi-polar, in order that the life-force may have instruments suitable for resistance, for conductivity and union, for sensibility and for associated sensibility. And yet, intricate and

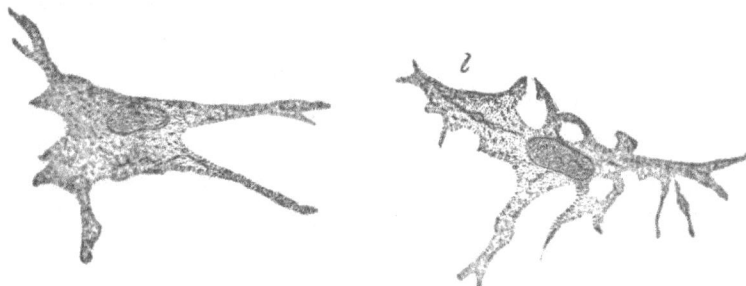

FIG. 6 (Quain, Fig. 64, vol. ii., p. 64).

complicated as the apparatus is, it is much less complex, as we shall be compelled to see immediately, than

the cerebro-spinal nervous mechanism, to be introduced for the expression or manifestation of life-purposes higher still than these.

Before, however, passing on to the cerebro-spinal nerve elements I introduce again, by the permission of Messrs Longmans, Green & Co., the Figure which is numbered 7 in this series.

This figure represents what is known as the Jelly of Wharton, and shows the structure of connective tissue at an early period of development. We see how it "consists of a pellucid jelly and nucleated corpuscles." "In the general course of development of the tissue, fibres, both white and elastic, are formed in the soft matrix, and finally obscure or obliterate this substance in a great measure." Other forms of connective tissue are formed in other ways, but this is a not uncommon mode of development.

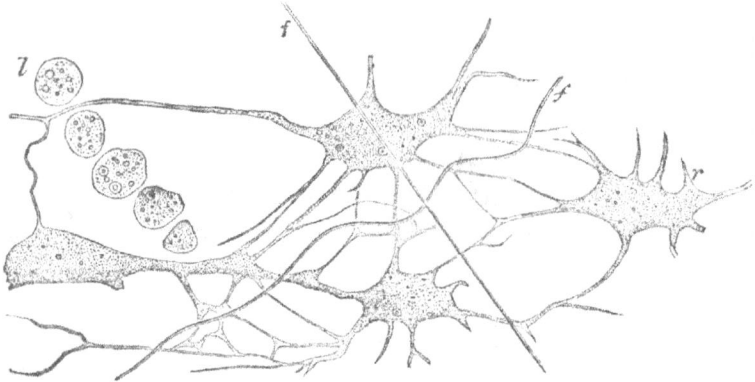

FIG. 7 (Quain, Fig. 71, vol. ii., p. 69).—JELLY OF WHARTON (RANVIER).

r, ramified cells intercommunicating by their branches; *l*, a row of leucocytes or migratory cells; *f.f.*, fibres coursing through the ground substance.

In order to show the differences between the structure of connective-tissue corpuscles and of cerebro-spinal nerve-cells, there is introduced here by permission of the publishers of Quain's "Elements of Anatomy," Figure 8 (in Quain, 144B, vol. ii., page 146).

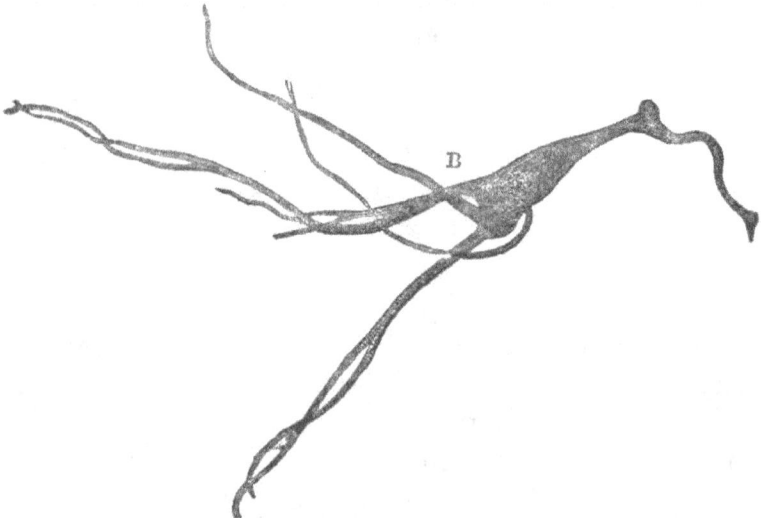

FIG. 8 (Quain, Fig. 144B, vol. ii., p. 146).

This figure represents a nerve-cell from the spinal cord, and we see how many poled it is, and are able perhaps to some extent to imagine how intricate and subtle must be the means of communication between parts when these parts are joined to others which communicate again with other cells. Thus we may see not only the means of sensibility and of associated sensibility, but also the means of appreciation of the same, and how the life-force proceeds to develop apparatus

for the manifestation of consciousness. This is still further shown from the representation of Figure 9 (Quain, No. 146, vol. ii., page 1447). Here we see the straight fibre *a*, the coiled fibre *b.b.*, with the smaller one *c.*, joining it. Both the last illustrations also show the cellular structure of the nervous elements. The cells can be seen with bounding membranes, protoplasmic contents, nucleus and nucleolus; and from these we may perhaps gain some impression of the manner in which the life-force proceeds to make for itself structures suitable for the exercise of consciousness in its lower and higher manifestations. Up to the present point, only the beginnings of the formation of these structures have been alluded to; but we see even at this stage, in

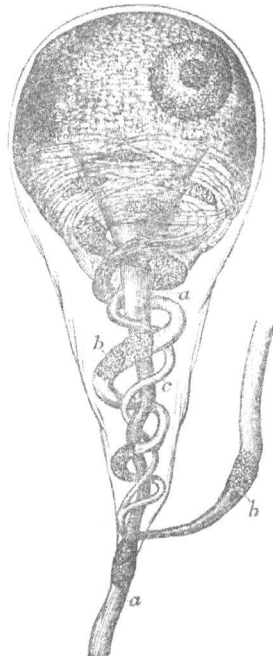

FIG. 9 (Quain, No. 146, vol. ii., p. 147).

the intricacy and complexity of the structure of the connective tissue itself, enough to occupy the mind in the attempt to understand the mechanism of response, conductivity, unity, sensibility and associated sensibility, even if we do not proceed further with the study (as happily we are not called upon at present to do) of the mechanism through which the higher powers of conscious response, conscious unity, conscious sensibility, and conscious association of sensibility are aspired to by the life-force and attained. It is a complicated mechanism, procreated by a force at first apparently quite unconscious, although later apparently it may rise to know what it is doing, to know that it knows, and perhaps even to know why it acts in these ways. And it may even become the instrument through which passive and unconscious operation rises into active and conscious co-peration with the design that is evolving the little world in which we dwell as part of that larger universe of which it forms a part.

V. PHYSIOLOGY OF THE CONNECTIVE TISSUES.

Although it has not been possible to keep quite separate the functions of the connective tissues from their structure, their physiology from their anatomy, still on the whole we have been occupied mainly with their anatomy, whether seen by the naked eye, or by microscopic examination. Having seen somewhat into that, we may now go on with a further inquiry into their functions or physiology

Besides the feelings of fatigue and aching which we experience when the connective tissues are congested, and the lightness and freedom felt when they are in proper condition, it is mainly through their functional action that we experience feelings of being well or of being ill, of activity and languor, of pain and pleasure, comfort and discomfort, of fitness and unfitness, and even, I think, of heat and cold. Generally speaking, these feelings are not localised or not definitely . I localised—— that is, we do not associate them with the affection of any particular part, although if any particular part of the connective tissues is specially congested or inflamed, as when we suffer from special peri-neuritis or neuralgia, or if any part of it inflames and suppurates, we may be compelled to do so. So striking indeed is the failure to localise many of these ailments that it is not infrequently the function of the medical adviser to inform patients that the seat of their pain is not in the place where they believe it to be. It sounds paradoxical to inform patients that their pain is not where they think it is; nevertheless, this is not infrequently the function of the medical adviser. And the reason for this is that the connective tissues are so universally distributed in the body, and each strand and cell of them are so inseparably connected with all the rest, that the localisation is lost or ill—defined; and so the feelings or sensations are general rather than particular. This is the

41

reason why young women, and sometimes older ones, burst out a-crying when their connective tissues are in this congested condition. They ache everywhere; they cannot localise the place or places of the ache; they are pained when they walk or move, and even some times when they eat or breathe, because the act of breathing puts ribs, muscles and joints and ligaments into action, and as all these parts are congested, or at least their coverings or envelopes are so, the simplest movements are painful, and the aching being general, life seems to be a burden, and the woman finds relief to her misery and helplessness in tears. It is barbarous to say that she has hysteria, and it is want of insight that makes us say that she is imagining it. We ought to direct her attention to the reason for her misery and to the causes that have led to the congestion of her connective tissues.

VI. THE FUNCTIONAL ACTION OF PARTS IS FELT RATHER THROUGH AFFECTION OF THE COVERINGS OF THE PARTS THAN THROUGH THE I INTIMATE STRUCTURE OF THE PARTS THEMSELVES.

It is a curious thing, but I think it is the case that, in the body generally, sensations and perceptions are not received by means of the functional action of the intimate structure of the parts most concerned so much as they are received through affection of the coverings of the parts. The feeling of resistance set up by muscular action is received through the functional action rather of the peri-mysium or covering of the muscles in action than through the affection of the intimate structure of the muscle itself. Neuralgia, or the pain we experience when certain nerves are affected, or when we think they are affected, or perhaps when we have been told they are affected, comes to us rather through affection of the covering of the nerve than through affection of the nerve itself. It is more commonly a perineuritis than a euritis, just as in the case of muscular affections it is rather a peri-mysitis which we experience than a mysitis. And the same is true, or very often is true, of sensations referred to bones. These are more often manifestations of periostitis than of osteitis-that is, they are more often affections of the bone-covering than of the bone itself. The same experience or similar experiences meet us when we investigate sensations referred to other organs, as the kidneys, the liver, the brain, the lungs. The sensations experienced, especially when painful, are rather expressions of distress in the coverings of the organs than in the organs themselves, from which it is apparent that the phenomena of initis are not unique in the body but form a particular case of a more general law. The connective tissues indeed follow the laws governing all other tissues in the body. They may be healthy, in which case we are almost unconscious of their existence; or they maybe congested, when their condition is a disturbance to us, either a conscious and localised disturbance, or an unlocalised and obscurely understood disturbance. Like other tissues, also, the connective tissues undergo congestion, inflammation, effusion, with or without resolution or absorption, suppuration and necrosis or local death. Not infrequently, after the congestion so commonly present has gone on for some time, we get an effusion of serum, clear or turbid, into a joint, a slight wrench or sprain or stumble seeming to be the immediate cause. And sometimes we see death of the part in bulk, when a portion of tendon or ligament, or even some of the mesh work of the connective tissue itself, may die and require to be slowly and painfully expelled from the body by sloughing, as when boils, or particularly carbuncles, appear in the body.

VII. RHEUMATISM.

WELL; I might have called these affections rheumatic. Rheumatism appears to me to be congestion or inflammation of connective tissue. It is initis. But the term rheumatism has come to be used in so undefined a way that I have thought it well to keep clear of it. In Greek ʹΡεῦμα means a stream, and is connected with the verb ῥέω, I flow; and the term rheumatism came to be applied to the pain felt when a discharge (as from the head, a running from the nose) suddenly ceased. The discharge, while it lasted, was a relief, or acted as a means of relieving the congestion of the mucous membrane of the nostrils and of its underlying connective tissue. With the cessation of the discharge, the aggravation of the congestion rose into pain. Of late, we have unfortunately complicated and confused our understanding of rheumatism by the inquiry as to its connection with the presence of uric acid in the blood and tissues. No doubt there are waste matters in the blood in the rheumatic condition, and no doubt uric acid is one of the most important of them; but scientifically and immediately rheumatism is congestion or other affection of the connective tissues. And as connective tissues are found everywhere in the body, as we have seen, to confine the name rheumatism to affections of synovial and serous membranes, as some authorities do, is to limit the use of the term too much; for, wherever connective tissue is found, there may be found congestion of it, and there may rheumatism therefore be found also.

The connective tissues not only form the coverings of nerves, bones and muscles, as well as the substance of ligaments and tendons, but they also form fasciae, as they are termed—that is, broad, firm layers surrounding muscles and bundles of muscles, from which muscular fibres spring and into which they are inserted. These can be well felt and seen on the outsides of the thighs forming the thick resistant tissues in these regions. These thick firm bands also send prolongations between the muscles, all these prolongations being connected with one another, and serving to separate muscles and sets or groups of muscles from one another. These can be particularly well seen if sections of muscular tissue are made, and in butchers' shops many of them can be seen on almost any day. The layers of connective tissue can be well seen, whiter than the redder muscular flesh, and passing in between the muscles, separating them one from another. Similar bands or membranes separate bundles or strands of nerves from others. They both separate them from one another and also join them to one another so as to allow them to act together. They both separate and unite. And not only do they separate muscle from muscle and nerve from nerve, but they also send processes or prolongations in between bundles of muscular tissue and of nervous tissue, so that the fibres of individual muscles and of individual nerves are separated from and joined to one another. These prolongations become finer and finer as the elements of muscle or of nerve become smaller and smaller. The prolongations are all connected with one another, and are continuous with one another, so that no particular portion of them can suffer without bringing sympathetic or conveyed suffering on the rest. From ligaments and tendons also pass prolongations to the bursae or little sacular diverticula connected with the origins and insertions of tendons, and generally close to joints. Prolongations even pass into the interiors of joints so that if ligaments or tendons are sprained or wrenched, not infrequently joints become affected also.

When we come to reflect that even the synovial linings of joints and the serous membranes generally, as found in the peritoneum lining the abdomen, in the pleurae covering the lungs, and in the membranes of the brain and spinal cord, both the internal membranes and the external membranes, are all laid or built upon connective tissue, underlying the plates of the serous membranes proper, we see what an exceedingly widespread distribution the connective tissue has. And we see therefore how numerous may be the symptoms, according as this, that or the other part of these widely distributed tissues is specially affected, and according as the affection of it, leaving one part may appear in another, either near or more remote from the part last affected. This accounts for the irregularity and erratic character of initis, and helps us to understand how, as it passes suddenly from one part to another, the patient may be suspected of exaggerating her symptoms or even of manufacturing them altogether. If the affection ceases in all parts at once and simultaneously, as sometimes it does, and then comes on again in one or more parts, the patient may be quite well at one time, and then suddenly, and apparently without cause, be very ill again at another; and so the onlooker may be tempted to think that the ailment is either unreal or needlessly exaggerated. Some patients no doubt do exaggerate their symptoms and some seem to become selfish and self-indulgent as if they even rejoiced in inflicting charges on their relatives in order to effect a cure. One can only say that judgment and common sense must be exercised in coming to a conclusion on such points. There are many little things that help us to come to a true conclusion; but if a young wife with three or four children dependent on her, or an older woman, spinster or married, complains of these obscure and irregular illnesses, and if her life-habits as to alcohol, etc., are correct, the probability is that the illness is a real one; and our aim ought to be to help her to a cure for the sake of husband and children as well as for her own.

VIII. THE URIC ACID THEORY OF RHEUMATISM.

The inquiry whether uric acid in the blood and tissues co-exists with the rheumatic state complicates the question by diverting attention from the state of the parts most immediately concerned.

The objection to the introduction of the inquiry whether uric acid is present in rheumatism, or connective-tissue congestion, or connective-tissue inflammation, and to the introduction of such a hybrid word as uric-acid-aemia, with its mixture of Greek and Latin, is that it complicates the issue. It takes a long time and requires a special analysis to determine if oxy-uri-chaemia is present or not; while we can say at once by the simplest examination if initis is present or not. The uric acid question is no doubt important, although rather as a particular case of a more general question than for its own sake only, since oxy-uri-chaemia is only one of the general signs of the catatribsemia or triphthaemia that is, of the presence of waste matters in the blood or tissues, or both, whether these find their way into the body through the digestion, or through breaking down of the tissues of the body, and their subsequent absorption by perversion of the function of nutrition (τρίβειν, to waste). Long before we can answer these questions, we can determine whether connective-tissue congestion is present, for mere pressure will enable us to answer the question yes or no. Besides that, uric acid is not the only poison which may be present in rheumatism, since we may have to do with lactic acid or butyric acid or other organic poisons. It is quite a question whether lactic acid may not be a more potent cause of rheumatism than uric acid, and distinguished men have held this view. But these questions require time and analysis to determine them, while whether initis is present or not can be answered at once.

IX. DIAGNOSIS.

As to diagnosis, the proof of the presence of initis is mostly clinical, but it is sufficient.

In the matter of diagnosis, I am often asked we can prove the reality of the existence of initis. Constantly do members of the medical profession say, "You cannot prove it." To this there are several replies, as we shall see. But the first comes in the form of asking the question, "Is clinical evidence then of no value?"Are we to believe that the great majority of patients who come to us ail nothing? Or that they are suffering from imaginary or alleged or put-on ailments? If a man says he aches, or if a woman complains of a headache or a backache, are we not to believe them? Who but themselves can tell whether they are suffering or not? No doubt it is often convenient for women and men (witness the excuses made by politicians and diplomatists about ill health) to say that they are ill when they are not. But are there no means of corroborating or of weakening the value of their statements? What about tenderness on pressure? Let the reader look at the photographs illustrating this book. Let him ask himself, or let her ask herself, if the tender places there shown exist, or if they do not? How often in the consulting-room have I said, when pointing out these tender places (for often their existence is quite unknown to patients whose only knowledge is that they feel ill), "Do you think that these places really ache, and do they really pain you when they are pressed upon, or do you think that you are being humbugged?" There is a universal "No, they are not unreal-they are not imaginary-they are real." Or a common answer is to the effect that whoever experiences these pains and tendernesses on pressure knows whether they are real or not.

One proof that the complaints are real is that some parts are felt to be much more tender than others. "I feel pressure here"—they will say— "but it is hardly painful, while pressure on that other part is very painful indeed." If the ailment was put on, it would probably be alleged to be equally painful at all places. I have known people, old and young, cry out when certain parts were pressed; and in the slow way in which the pain disappears, the onlooker can almost see the invisible motion which is affecting the pained connective tissues at one point after another, until, in course of time, it quiets down and subsides; and the patient gets ease again. Is it to be believed that all this is not real? If a man is carving a joint at the dinner-table, and if he lays down the knife and fork because his arms ache so that it is uncomfortable for him to go on with what he is doing-is it credible that there is no cause for his behaviour? And if on pressure at the inner elbows and on the muscles of the fore-arms and on the neck of the radius, he complains of tenderness and pain, are we not to believe him? "Oh," says the critic, "it has not been demonstrated to exist by microscopic examination." Well I but should we be justified in excising some of the connective tissue in order to make a microscopic examination of it? Even in that case we might or might not find the congestion of which we were in search. Patients very rarely die in this condition, and when they do die of other diseases (often consequences of this preceding condition, though not generally considered to be so) the connective tissue is not examined microscopically with a view to saying whether it is congested or not. My impression is that the infiltration of the tissue corresponding to the aching complained of would not infrequently be found if it were looked for. But the clinical evidence is to me so complete and irrefragable and so convincing that I do not think it necessary to ask for further evidence nor do I think we should be justified in asking leave to excise portions of the connective tissue in order to prove whether it was congested or not. And if we did make the painful experiment we might or might not succeed in determining the point at issue. The interference with vital action caused by our experiment might easily vitiate our whole conclusion.

In some cases death has occurred in the acute stage of rheumatic synovitis, or what is often called rheumatic fever. And in some of these cases, although microscopic search was made, no congestion has been found in the synovial membrane lining the joint examined. Are we to be asked to believe that the patient screaming out with the excruciating pain of such a condition had no justification for his complaint at all? Is it likely that there was no congestion, even if temporary, when the pain was so severe? In other inflammatory conditions there is throbbing felt by the patient and detectable by the examiner's finger. Is it not likely that a similar congestion is present in synovitis? And yet it might be so fugitive as to be undemonstrable. There are other sorts of evidence as well as microscopic evidence. Is it not well known that in many cases of acute synovitis, or rheumatic fever, the pain suddenly leaves one joint, say the knee, to appear almost immediately in another, say the hip? We should probably fail, therefore, to demonstrate the presence of congestion in the former if we looked for it, and in the case of the latter we might or might not be able to demonstrate it either.

The limits of experiment in the living subject are much narrower because the facts are much more complicated than they are in what we call inanimate nature. The antivivisection controversy has up to the present time raged around the question whether experiments were justifiable on the lower animals in order that benefit might accrue to human beings. There are wide differences of opinion on that question, as we know. But I venture to think that if any scientific inquirer were to propose to carry out painful experiments on human beings in order to determine such a question as whether the microscope shows the presence of visible blocking or congestion of the connective tissues in rheumatism, he would very soon find out the universal horror that would be set up by his proposal. And there are other considerations which arise when we investigate the phenomena of living beings with which I do not deal; but I may say that they depend mainly on this, that the scientific and undisputed facts are always capable of many and different interpretations, and as each of us forms, and indeed must form, his own interpretations, there is room for very considerable difference of view as to the interpretation of the facts.

The clinical evidence is to me overwhelming. Corns are overgrowths of the outer part of the skin which is called epithelium. But corns are often found along with the swellings of toe-joints so frequently found in elderly persons, and which, often associated with overgrowth of the nails, are termed gouty or rheumatic. Not infrequently ulceration is also present. The enlargement and distortion of the joints is unmistakable when it appears. In fact it is often permanent and never got rid of again. But coincidently with the thickening of the epithelial part of the skin and of the nails so often present along with corns, there is often present a congestion of the inner part of the skin where it is loosely and yet firmly held in its place by the underlying connective tissue; and that thickening again is coincident with the general thickening which has ended in the enlargement of the joint. Sometimes, indeed, though happily not very often, destruction of the joint by suppuration and necrosis or death of a portion of the bone occurs, and amputation has to be resorted to. To doubt the diagnosis in face of evidence of this kind, which no man of experience can have failed to encounter, seems to me to be carrying criticism to the point of utter scepticism, Pyrrhonism and futility; and I must say that I think that those who do so have not considered the question with sufficient care.

For a long time before such a necessity as amputation of a limb or portion of it has been forced on us, the obscure achings and pains referred to have been going on. They have often gone on for years before. They were indeed warnings and premonitions of what was to come, which, had they been attended to in time, might have enabled us so to advise the patient that he might have saved his great toe or his knee, to take two cases which occur to me as I write. I am sure that it is very often because we fail to see the significance of these obscure symptoms, and to attend to them in time, that such disasters happen from time to time in practice. There are other consequences also of the slowly accumulating congestion of connective tissue that arise from time to time. These will be dealt with more fully later (see pp. 78 - 80), but I will say here only this about them, that although their connection with a long continued (or chronic) initis is seldom recognised, it is, I believe, very real. Thus such disasters as apoplexy, the onset of Bright's disease, and cancer, not to mention that of slow crippling rheumatism and gout, are very often preceded by the signs and symptoms which we are considering. And, of course, the important practical consideration is that, had sufficient notice been taken of the preceding and curable conditions, the subsequent incurable ones would either not have occurred, or they would probably have been postponed for many years. It is a serious and a very practical question whether these incurable conditions arise after the long and slow occurrence of initis in the body, and whether therefore their onset might not be prevented for an indefinite length of time. I at least have no doubt how this question should be answered.

X. FURTHER CONSIDERATIONS REGARDING THE FUNCTIONS OF THE CONNECTIVE TISSUES.

I HAVE said that the connective tissue is the organ of common sensibility—that is, that it is the organ through which we feel well or ill, fit for work or unfit, etc. Another way of stating this proposition would be to say that the connective tissues are the common sensorium (sensorium commune) or common sensory of the body. This seems to me to be a very illuminating proposition from the psychological point of view, but for the moment it must be left to be dealt with by each reader for himself, the caution being always kept in mind that common sensibility and the appreciation of common sensibility are probably functional expressions of different organs (connective-tissue and cerebro-spinal nerve-tissue).

But the connective tissue is also, I believe, the organ through which we feel *warm* or *cold*; and through which also we have the feeling of *resistance* when pressing against a weight, as in lifting when the weight is moved; or when our power is insufficient to move it and when resistance only is experienced. Of course, it is not the organ of the special senses, as of seeing and hearing, although even as regards these, and also as regards its functions in touch or tactile sensibility, a good deal could be said which cannot be dealt with now. The reader will, however, probably think that reasons should be advanced for what is now being said, since many believe that common sensibility is the function rather of the nervous system than of the connective tissues. I have, however, I hope, somewhat anticipated this objection and criticism in reminding readers of the cells which are found in the connective tissues, and in depicting the structures from an authoritative source. If the function of the connective tissue is generally considered to be only that of uniting the various parts of the body and of conducting impressions from one part to another (unity and conductivity) this is to narrow too much the function of this important structure, since it takes account only of the fibres, white, yellow or elastic, of which it is mainly composed, but takes no account of the cells which also enter into its composition. While all parts of the body respond to stimuli, and manifest therefore what may be called the apamoebic or responsive quality, the force of animal life so arranges things, or it so works, that each tissue responds in accordance with its special structure.

I do not wish to use the ordinary expression that the constitution of an organ or of a tissue determines its properties or that its connections determine its functions, because this seems to imply that the force depends on the thing, that the power depends on the instrument. I see no evidence that this is so. In fact, it seems to me that it would be nearer the truth to say that the force (of animal life—e.g. zoo-dynamic) determines the constitution of the tissue which shall be fit to do that which the animal life-force unconsciously wishes to accomplish—that is, if I *have* to choose between the two views, I prefer the view that the need to function determines the constitution of the structure fit to be the means of carrying out the function, before the view which holds that constitution determines properties and connections determine functions. All that science shows is that constitution, property and function are always co-ordinate and co-related to one another. Which one is the cause of the other, or whether either is the cause of the other, is not a scientific but a philosophic question. In fact, constitution and property, structure and function, arise simultaneously and no doubt are common or simultaneous effects of a common cause (the action of the force of animal life or zoo-dynamic) rather than cause and effect of one another.

Purpose and plan appear to be visible in all the actions of animal life-force or zoo-dynamic. To say that zoo-dynamic is apparently unconscious of the plan that guides it may be to use the language of paradox, but is nevertheless true. The horse which pulls a cart zigzag up a hill unconsciously takes the direction of least resistance, and that which is most in harmony with the comfort of its life, although it has never studied physics, nor has it the capacity to do so. The bicyclist acts similarly in similar circumstances, and may or may not know anything of physics either. It is even a moot point whether the bicyclist climbs the hill any better for having studied physics than if he knows nothing about the composition of forces, although no doubt he experiences a much higher form of satisfaction if he does know. Unconscious plan therefore seems to have more to be said for it than at first sight appears possible. The truth seems therefore to be that the need to take the direction of least resistance, and the introduction of the apparatus necessary for this, arise in the developing organism simultaneously, as effects of the force of animal life which is the cause of both. They are therefore simultaneous effects of a common cause and not cause and effect of one another. And similarly the existence of organs, their structure and properties and functions, are seen to be co-ordinated or concomitant effects of the various forms of life-force. This view applies not only to the connective tissues, but also to all other organs, as the liver with its bile secretion, the kidneys with their excretion, the brain, the lungs and the rest. As the force of life requires them, they arise or are procreated simultaneously, the organs and their functions at once, not as cause and effect of one another, but as concomitant effects of their common cause.

To say that the connective tissues connect every part of the body with every other is to give them a high place in function, since this is only another way of saying that they are the structures used by the force of life to act as the means by which the feeling of unity or solidarity shall be experienced in the animal body. (The same considerations no doubt apply to the phenomena of plant-life or phyto-dynamic, but our consideration is at present confined to the facts of animal life or zoo-dynamic. The force of life in general, including plants and animals, I call bio-dynamic—but indeed all nature is alive to a lesser or greater extent.) It is by the functional action of the connective tissues that we know without being told, and without requiring to be told, that every part of the body, however unimportant it may seem, belongs to the body and forms part and parcel of it. We realise this often in a surprising way, if a small part like, say, the little finger happens to be inflamed, for when this is so, every movement, however slight, sets up pain, not only in the part immediately affected, but also in remote parts that we perhaps imagined had little or no connection with it. Yet every slight movement of the small inflamed part seems to jar the whole body.

Analogies may probably arise in the reader's mind between the behaviour of the body physical and that of the body political and social. If it is through the action of the connective tissues that the unity of the body physical is effected, is not the body political held together and unified by the bonds of good will that ought to be developed throughout it? And if we find disturbances taking place in the body political, jars and wranglings and strikes, is not this probably because the bonds of good will are becoming blocked, plugged and choked by self-interest or class-interest, just as the connective tissues so often get into a similar state by over-nutrition? If individuals and groups of individuals in the State seek their own interests unduly, the State must feel disturbances just like those felt in the body by irritation or inflammation of the connective tissues. The aching of the little finger acting as a source of jar to the whole body is paralleled by over-indulgence in self-interest by individuals or classes in the

State. Even in the congested state of the connective tissues which is so much commoner than that of inflammation, the effect is to render the movements of the body slow and heavy, if they are not exactly painful. But when congestion becomes inflammation, then positive pain generally sets in. And so in the body political. If the self-interest of individuals or of persons or classes in the state is over-indulged, the body political is oppressed, and movement -that is, progress— is slow, heavy and sluggish. But if the class feeling is still stronger, then disputes and contentions cause such disturbances as to amount to pain or revolution.

The superficial observer of the body physical may perhaps see only that the connective tissues are thickened and may be disposed to view that thickening as a sign of increased strength, in place of the diminished responsiveness and the diminished strength and fitness which it really indicates. And the superficial observer of the body political, seeing only the immediate improvement in individual or in class interests, may not inquire at what cost to the general well—being such individual or class benefits have been attained. But the onset of apoplexy or of cancer in the one case, or the occurrence of social revolution in the other, may open our eyes too late to the insidious nature of the causes which for a long time had been choking up the connective tissues of the body physical, or blocking the subtle and delicate bands and bonds of good will in the body political.

The reader may, if he chooses to, pursue this analogy further, and may perhaps see how so many fair organisms have been too early destroyed and how so many fine states have been destroyed, and how if such causes continue in the present and the future, they cannot fail to be followed by like effects. The order of the universe in which we live permits of no other issue.

XI. FUNCTIONS OF CONNECTIVE-TISSUE CELLS AND OF NERVE-CELLS. A GENERAL VIEW OF THE RELATIONS OF FUNCTION TO STRUCTURE.

I NEED not repeat here what has already been said when considering the functions of the cells of the connective tissues and comparing them with those exercised through the nerve-cells. The net result is that to have an impression is not by any means necessarily the same thing as to know that we have it, since we may receive an impression through the unconscious functioning of one set of structures, while we may know that we receive it through the (still unconscious) use of another. We may become conscious co-workers with the forces whose harmonious co-operation keeps agoing the universe in which we live, and of which our planet, and the sun which lights and warms it, makes only a very small part. Our individual lives are only like the drops of water whose will-less and unconscious aggregation makes the mighty river of life; and to understand this seems to be one of the highest functions of humanity. What complication of the organic mechanism, what intricacy of arrangement of structure may be demanded, or what ascending hierarchy of organic forms may require to arise, in order that the human life-force may be able to perform, and to be conscious of performing, this noble function, would form one of the most difficult, though at the same time perhaps the most fascinating and entrancing, of all studies.

But there is a gradation even now plainly visible in the little examination which we have made into the matter. And we find response manifested through all tissues; we find conductivity and unity manifested through the introduction of fibres and bands; we find sensibility manifested through cells with their walls, their protoplasmic contents, their nuclei and nucleoli;

we find associated sensibility manifested when poles or processes reach the processes of other cells still higher in the scale of organisation; and sensibility of sensibility of sensibility before consciousness is reached through the adaptation of the organic mechanism to it. And how long the chain or how intricate is the mechanism that is introduced by anthropino-zoo-dynamic before conscious co-working with the forces of the universe is attained we do not know, because the arrangements elude even our most subtle means of investigation. But it seems very probable that the same processes of mal-assimilation, and especially of over-nutrition, which block the coarser fibres and cells of the connective tissues and so render them less efficient for the animal-life purposes, may very easily so choke up as entirely to destroy the functions of the fine connecting poles which join nerve-cell to nerve-cell, and thus may interfere with the function of sensibility of sensibility of sensibility. And of course sensibility of sensibility of sensibility may be prevented, and so the high consciousness of co-working, and the desire therefor, may be indefinitely postponed. No doubt in the evolution of humanity this altitude (or higher) will be attained, but we may have to reflect that our individual opportunity of doing so may have to be attained through our conscious exertion, and that if it is missed it may not recur.

XII PELIOSIS

THE fibres of the connective tissue, being thus the organ of unity and conductivity, may be stronger or weaker. They may have, as scientific men often express it, more or less resistance. In some cases they are very strong, firm and elastic, and will bear a great deal of strain without giving way, while in others they give way easily, and even tear or rupture partially or completely under comparatively little strain. Inequality of resistance is no doubt the direct gift of life in many cases—that is, as human beings differ in degrees of force and strength in every human way, and as all of us do not come into the world with equal degrees of resisting power in any direction, so do we show differing degrees of strength or resistance in connective tissues. (See pages 69 to 71.)

XIII. ARE DIFFERENCES IN RESISTING POWER TO BE ASCRIBED TO HEREDITY ?

THESE differences are often attributed to inheritance. But a better way of viewing the facts appears to be to consider that the force of human animal life (anthropino-zoo-dynamic) as it comes from an infinite source (being in fact one of the forces, or one variety of the forces, whose aggregate makes the universal omnipotent and eternal energy by which all things do consist) gifts or endows its human procreations and incarnations with an infinite variety of degrees of life-force. The marvel would be if it did not. If we found any two leaves exactly alike or any two animals or any two human beings or any two faces or any two pairs of eyes or other features, and if this was a very frequent occurrence, we might readily believe that we were studying the effects of a limited power. But the absolutely unpredictable number of varieties of resistance and of other qualities and combinations of qualities makes us feel the omnipotence and infinity of the force (always within its own order, of course) with which we have to deal. I have no doubt that the true explanation of this is that the life-force itself comes from an infinite source; that it is one of the varieties of the one universal energy. Each observer will form his own conclusion on this point. But our idea of inheritance is modified by our view.

Inheritance or heredity, as commonly viewed, is, I suppose, the receipt of qualities *from* ancestors. But what if it should turn out to be, not this, but merely the condition of qualities at birth gifted to organisation by the force of life acting through ancestors? If heredity comes *from* ancestors, what gave the qualities *to* the ancestors? Did the ancestors receive them from their ancestors in turn? Or how did the original ancestors come by them? Evidently they must have begun to appear at some time. Otherwise, the strain of organisation, human or other, must have been on this planet from the beginning. Neither scientific men, however, nor the laity, seem to think this probable, for they speak of the origin of life, and indeed even of the origin of our planet itself and of the comparatively small solar system to which it belongs. There is a very simple explanation, it seems to me, of the eternity of matter (if it *were* or *is* eternal)—namely, that matter is the continuous procreation of the infinite eternal and omnipotent energy by which all things do consist. This energy procreates matter, always has done so and always will, so far as we can see.

XIV. IS MATTER ETERNAL IN DURATION OR EXTENT?

THE eternity of matter is on this view a derived eternity. It is derived from the eternal energy by which all things do consist. But this eternal energy is itself also derived from the only source adequate to account for it. And, in point of fact, eternal energy constantly emanating from the Infinite is constantly procreating matter. Matter is constantly wasting, through the action on it of the energy which procreated and procreates it, since material substance cannot bear the action of energy without wasting and withering and being consumed by it. No doubt there are compensations for this, since the light and heat of kinetic energy illuminate and warm dark and cold places, coincidently with the waste of material substance. Along with the wasting of matter, the universe is lighted and warmed—which reflection may perhaps console the evanescent passenger through life and show him how his passing may contribute to the evolution of the universe in which he lives. The process will continue whether we appreciate it or not, but how much better will it be if we can rise to the conscious realisation of it. The constant movement of matter, the ebb and flow of its tides, the rise and fall in alternation of its behaviour, if it impresses us with belief in its solidity and permanence on the one hand, impresses us still more with belief in its evanescence and intermittence on the other. And the intermittent waste and repair of matter through the action of kinetic energy on it is the effect of the inability of matter to bear the action of this continuous energy. Under this action matter wastes and must be repaired, and also rested, if it is to become fit to respond again to the action of kinetic energy. Waste, repair and rest in so-called inanimate things, and waste, repair and sleep in so called animate nature (but is not all nature alive or animate, more or less?), account for the intermittent

64

qualities shown by matter when it is responding to the action of the continuous action of the continuous energy of the universe. The eternity of matter, then, on this view (if it *were* or *is* eternal), is, first derived from energy which is constantly reprocreating it as it wastes; but, second, it is apparent only and not real, since matter is. constantly vanishing; but as constantly as matter is being wasted in this way and "vanishing without return" (G. le Bon) as constantly is energy reprocreating it. In this way the universe, which would otherwise have become void and empty generations ago, or eternities ago, by the vanishing of matter, remains constantly full, through the action of the eternal energy which is for ever emanating from its infinite and eternal source. Matter and energy may thus both seem to be eternal, but the eternity of matter is, first, derived (from energy) and, second, it is apparent only and not real. The eternity, infinity and omnipotence of energy is also derived (from the Infinite) but, second, it is real because it is for ever emanating from its Infinite, Eternal and Omnipotent Source, the Divine Himself. And being infinite, and untrammelled by space and time, the Infinite so works that matter and energy are simultaneous and successive, although both simultaneousness and succession are expressions allowable only because of the weakness and blindness of the limited faculties of observers striving to comprehend the universe in which we live and move and have our being.

This explanation of the universe, while it is an explanation, so far as it goes, can never be a comprehension by a finite mind of infinite working. But it is so simple, and at the same time so comprehensive and satisfying, that I am compelled to accept it although, of course, each observer must form his own opinion and conclusion on the matter. At any rate, the fact remains that there is a vast variety of degrees of resistance found in the connective tissues which hold together the bodies of human beings both at the time they come into the world at birth, and also later in life when various other conditions have affected them. These varying conditions could easily be measured, say, by the differing amounts of weight which could be lifted or moved by muscles and their connective-tissue coverings of varying degrees of strength. Some tissues would become peliotic from rupture of the connective tissue and its accompanying fine vessels on raising or moving weights of a less amount, while other connective tissues would not yield or give way on being made to move or raise much heavier weights. The conditions found at birth are usually considered to be hereditary, while those found later in life are considered to be acquired. To consider the former as the sum of the facts at birth, and the latter as the sum of the facts at any given period of life, would be a more accurate and less theoretical method of viewing them, and at the same time simpler and less confusing, since we should be confining ourselves more to facts—that is, to science— and striving to keep clear of theories to explain the facts—that is, striving to keep clear of philosophy. And the plain fact is, that the resistance of the connective tissues of the body varies very much both in infants coming into the world, and also at different periods of their life-history.

Evidently inheritance does not explain these differences at birth, because inherited conditions themselves vary as much as any other life–quality from generation to generation to generation; and the children of delicate parents often show much resistance, while the children of stronger parents are often endowed with less resistance. Also different children of the same parents show different degrees of resistance. And if on the ordinary view (if indeed there is an ordinary or generally accepted view) qualities may be accumulated from generation to generation, surely a minor degree of these qualities might, nay, must, have been conferred on an ancestral form at some time in what seems to us the long period during which our race has been on this planet. Length of duration in time and extension in space are, however, human conceptions from whose dominion it is hardly possible for us to escape, but they have no relation whatever to an infinite power. I have no doubt myself that the races of plants and animals, lower and human, appeared, when the environment was ready for them, by simultaneous succession or by simultaneous appearance, and not by successive succession—that is, that they appeared, each species of them (and possibly a number of varieties and species)—together at once and simultaneously—that is, old and mature and young and infantile and unborn at once and simultaneously, and not under the appearance of a single ancestor or ancestral pair at all.

How the human mind ever came to limit the working of infinite and omnipotent power by the mean and inadequate conception that required it to incarnate itself in a common ancestor or in a pair of common ancestors, from which in turn were to be developed all the varieties and individuals that are seen in nature, is a mystery which appears insoluble—unless, indeed, it be because we insensibly assume that infinite power is under the same limitations as bind us down. Of course, it is a question of evidence; but the evidence, though it takes account, and must take account, of variation, seems to have taken too little account of mutation and of the sudden appearance of new forms whose ancestors do not seem altogether to account for them.

XV. INSTANCES OF SIMULTANEOUS SUCCESSION OR OF THE SIMULTANEOUS APPEARANCE OF WHAT USUALLY OCCUR AS SUCCESSIVE PHENOMENA IN NATURE.

THERE are in nature many instances of the simultaneous appearance of two or more structures when the environment is ready for them. This seems to be the method of development of the protozoa, in which protoplasmic elements, fine bounding membranes, spores, bacilli and mycelium all appear at once and simultaneously. But in the development of the higher organisms many similar experiences are met with also. Thus we read in Quain's "Anatomy": "The first red-blood corpuscles are formed very early in embryonic life, simultaneously with and in the interior of the first blood-vessels" (vol.ii.,p.34). And in the same way we may watch the development of the blood-vessels and of the lymphatic vessels simultaneously, plexuses of lymphatics surrounding the blood-vessels, and blood-vessels supplying the lymphatics, and both appearing together. The blood and blood-vessels are formed simultaneously, not the vessels first, to carry the blood and then the blood to be carried; nor yet the blood first and then vessels to convey it, but simultaneously, as if to show (what is no doubt the case) that the blood and the blood-vessels are simultaneous effects of a common cause—viz. the life-force (zoo-dynamic) whose place in the manifestation of the universal energy we have already seen. Similarly the blood-vessels arise simultaneously with the lymphatic vessels, not blood-vessels first to receive the lymph from the lymphatic system and then lymphatic vessels to convey the lymph into the blood-vessels; nor yet lymphatics first to pass the lymph into the blood-vessels; and then blood-vessels to receive the lymph; but both simultaneously. Successive succession, as the succession of day on night or of son on father, are instances from which it is quite plain what Nature's methods of working are. It is easier to see that day and night are successive effects of a common cause than perhaps it is to see that structure and function are concomitant effects of their common cause.

But an attempt to understand these things might have kept the scientific mind straight when it found its way either into philosophy or into attempts to account for origins. As, however, none of us were there to see (and, if we had been, could we have comprehended?) each of us must form his own conclusion. It is however something to have seen that in nature, structure or constitution, and function or use arise together and simultaneously, since we are so apt to imagine either that structure is the cause of function or that the need to function is the procreator of the structure through which the function is to be performed. As structure and function arise together, the containing vessels and the contained blood, the blood-vessels to receive the lymph and the lymphatics to pass the lymph on; the hepatic structure simultaneously with the secretion of bile through it; the construction of the nervous system and brain as the instruments of thought, and the occurrence of thinking through them at once and simultaneously, we see plainly that neither is structure the cause of function, nor is the need to function the cause of the introduction of the structure through which function shall be performed; but that the true view is that structure and the need to function are concomitant effects of a common cause—viz. in this case no doubt the force of human life or anthropino-zoo-dynamic, a variety or one of the forces whose aggregate makes the universal energy by which all things do consist.

When the conducting and unifying connective-tissue fibres are weak, and little resistant, they easily tear and give way under strain, and as the finest blood-vessels and lymphatic ducts go along with them, the blood-vessels rupture along with the connective tissues, and when they do so, they bleed under the skin and form black and blue marks visible enough to the unaided vision. This is intelligible enough when the rupture is caused by some violent wrench or strain. The part becomes black and blue, or peliotic, as it is called (πελιός, purple). As we watch it, in course of time it becomes green, then yellow, and finally disappears. It is easy to understand this when accident or strain accounts for the peliosis. It is more of a puzzle when there is no wrench or strain to account for the peliosis. But really there is no difficulty, because in some people the connective tissues are so weak and non-resistant that they give way and rupture with no wrench at all, in the mere act of moving or walking or even breathing. And of course when they do so, the ruptured fine vessels bleed under the skin and show discolorations similar to those produced by the more violent wrenches or sprains which would affect any one, however strong may be his connective tissues.

This peliotic condition has been known for a very long time. Hippocrates wrote about it some 2400 years ago, and very likely it was known to his predecessors. I am not aware whether its cause has been explained before, but it is very easy to see that excessive friability of the connective tissues is an adequate cause, and no doubt it is the real one. How very weak these tissues become in some cases is indeed almost incredible. The merest trifle of movement of the parts affected will suffice to rupture them sometimes, and occasionally rupture seems to occur without any movement at all, or without more than the simplest movement which anyone ought to be able to effect without discomfort. We see people not infrequently (especially women, no doubt, but sometimes men show the same phenomena) on whose bodies, or parts like the arms, if we lay a hand, with however gentle a grasp, the signs of the grasp appear the next day or the day after, with the black and blue marks of the fingers. Sometimes hurrying to catch a train is enough to set up these marks and sometimes even the act of breathing seems sufficient to do it and to cause peliotic marks about the chest or elsewhere in the body.

Now in considering the real as distinguished from the imaginary nature of the affections of the connective tissues we shall be very unwise to neglect or ignore objective conditions such as these. Complaints of pain for which we can find no adequate cause may be so subjective that it may be difficult to determine if they are real or not. But peliosis is objective. The observer can see it for himself, whether the patient draws attention to it or not. Its existence forms, on the whole, the most powerful argument in favour of the real, as distinguished from the imaginary, nature of the ailment, the initis or connective-tissue congestion with weakness, from which so many persons suffer.

XVI. FORMATION OF WEALS ON THE SKIN.

I OUGHT to mention here another objective sign frequently observed in persons suffering in these ways. If, in such persons, we draw the finger-nail lightly along the skin anywhere, say about the chest or arms, almost immediately there appear red lines or weals on the skin in the tracks along which the nail has passed. This shows the congestion and weakness or lowered resistance of the outer part of the skin, its epithelial part, and is no doubt coincident with congestion of the deeper layer also. It is of course an objective fact which can be made out by the observer and is not at all dependent on the statement of the patient. In fact, patients often enough are not aware of the existence of so much susceptibility until their attention has been directed to it.

XVII. IS THE CONNECTIVE TISSUE THE ORGAN THROUGH WHICH WE FEEL HEAT AND COLD ?

THE connective tissue being thus, as has been seen, the organ of unity or solidarity and of conductivity, and there being reason to think that it is the organ of general response, or the common sensory; is it, it may be further asked, also the organ through which heat and cold are felt? It is probably the organ through which we feel well or ill, fit for work or unfit, comfortable and happy or uncomfortable and miserable. The reasons for suggesting that it is in addition the organ through which sensations of heat and cold are perceived through the bodily structure are these: On laying the hand on any part of the body, either our own body or that of others, it feels warm or cold, as the case may be, in contrast with the examining hand, warm if the hand is cold, cold if the hand is warm. This is the first impression, but if we examine further, we find that some of the deeper parts vary very much from the superficial ones in the amount of warmth which is suggested through them to the examiner's hand. If the hand is laid on the calf of the leg, the first impression generally is that it is cold. But if we let the hand rest say over the course of the soleus muscle along the inner edge of the shin-bone, a different impression is often received, for there the limb may be warm or hot.

If this experience does not justify us in saying that the connective tissue is the organ of thermo-taxis or heat arrangement in the body, it at least shows, or seems to show, that it may be the organ through which the heat of the body is distributed or localised—i.e. that it is the thermo-topic organ? Warmth or heat is one of the invariable qualities of kinetic or active energy. In this case no doubt it is a quality of animal-life energy (zoo-dynamic) or of human-life energy (anthropino-zoo-

73

dynamic), but it is distributed by material changes in the organism, or rather, let us say, concurrently with the occurrence of material changes in the organism. Similar experiences may often occur as regards the feeling of warmth or cold communicated to the hand of the observer when examining other parts of the body, as, e.g., the head and neck of a patient. Often we may find the forehead cold and the back of the neck hot. Sometimes both are hot, and sometimes the neck may be cold and the forehead hot, although this is not so common an experience as the other. But these facts seem to go towards corroborating the view that sensations of heat and cold arise through affections of the connective tissues, even if the appreciation of them is received through the use of the nervous system (often enough an unconscious use).

Then the relations of the connective tissues to the organs of touch through which we have experiences of heat and cold as well as of tactile sensibility seem to me to suggest the same conclusion to the mind. There is not space to deal with this adequately, and I do not say that it is proved, but it seems likely that the connective tissues are the thermo-topic organ in the body even if they are not the thermo—taxic organ. And this likelihood seems to be strengthened by the reflection that when the feverish state sets in, and when the heat distribution and the heat liberation in the body are most emphatically interfered with, the accompanying aching in head, back and limbs is evidently associated with physiological changes in the connective tissues of the body. But all these considerations seem to lead to the conclusion, or at least the suggestion, that the connective tissues are the organ through which impressions of heat and cold are received (thermotopia and psychro-topia), as well as of unity and common sensibility or general aesthesia or zesthesis ($\alpha\H\iota\sigma\theta\eta\sigma\iota s$).

XVIII. THE RELATIONS BETWEEN THE CONNECTIVE TISSUE AND THE LYMPH.

WE have already seen that the connective tissue may be considered to be the largest secreting gland in the body, since it secretes the lymph which forms a bulk of two or three times as much as that of the blood. Further, the lymphatic glands through which the lymph is elaborated and rendered more corpuscular are also embedded in the connective tissue. Now, when we reflect that the lymphatic system, originating thus in the connective tissue, has for its function the expression or squeezing out from the blood of its watery parts containing any excess of nutriment greater than the requirements of the tissues, and so passing it to the lymphatic glands which fit it for conveyance back again to the blood for re-use in the economy, it is evident that we are in presence of facts of the very highest significance in nutrition.

There is no lymphatic system, it may be observed, in the invertebrates. The blood-vessels of the invertebrata convey a colourless or nearly colourless blood, and no lymphatic vessels are inserted by the invertebrate force of life because none are required in the comparatively low form of organisation and the comparatively coarse form of nutrition to which invertebrate animals have attained. But that the lymphatic system, when it exists, has for its function the reconveyance to the blood of nutritive material not used in the circulation of the blood to the tissues is evident from several considerations. And the chief one is this, that the lymphatic ducts, after conveying their contents to the lymphatic glands, pass on to join the thoracic duct and then to fall, as to their larger portion, into the great vein at the root of the neck on the left side. And the great significance of this arrangement becomes apparent when we remember that the thoracic duct is the channel by which the white particles of digested food, called chyle, are conveyed from the small intestine and emptied into the veins for the enrichment of the blood through the processes of digestion.

It would be impossible in the space at our disposal to describe minutely the processes through which food passes in digestion; nor indeed is it necessary for present purposes to do more than remember that the chyle of the small intestine, to which the food has been converted in digestion, enters the thoracic duct, which conveys its contents to the blood at the left side of the neck, and that on its way the thoracic duct receives the contents of the lymphatic system which are thus passed as a mixed whole into the blood for its enrichment. The lymphatics of the right side of the head and right upper part of the body pass by a smaller duct into the venous blood at the root of the right side of the neck. In these ways all the contents of the lymphatic system are passed into the blood, and as they join the thoracic duct which contains the digestive products proper, the connection of the lymphatic system with the digestion becomes apparent. It is quite plain in fact that the lymphatic system forms the apparatus of a complementary digestive process. It is very important that we should bear this in mind, because an essential part of right treatment depends on it. For when the connectives tissue takes on the state of initic congestion, it is because its texture has become congested and blocked with waste materials, and this happens because digestion has been imperfectly performed.

Now the commonest cause of this imperfect digestion or assimilation is the fact that too much food has been taken into the body; and so we see how one of the most important means of treatment is restriction of the diet. Obviously if too much food has passed in and has caused indigestion in consequence, one of the means of rectifying this must be to allow to pass in only as much as can be assimilated. It will be necessary to refer to this again. But in the meantime we have incidentally cleared up a good deal of the obscurity attaching to the condition of initis, and have come to realise how that obscurity accounts for the large number of different names given to the affection. These are of two sorts, (1st) functional names dependent on symptoms described by the patients; and (2nd) anatomical names dependent on the parts affected or supposed to be affected. And there are (3rd) mixed names, perhaps the most numerous of all, connected with both of these factors. Thus we find the name neurasthenia, or weakness of nerves, often given to it. Sometimes it is called neurosis or nervousness (both of these names implying that it is the nerves that are affected rather than the coverings as we have seen to be the ease). Then it is called hysteria or wombiness, which of course cannot apply to men, although they often suffer from the disease quite as much as women (ὕστερον, womb). Then it is called general debility, a purely symptomatic and functional name. Sometimes it is called by the mixed name of rheumatic neuralgia and sometimes by that of neuralgic rheumatism, names which no doubt it is often convenient to use, since patients *will* have their diseases named, some of them seeming to prefer to have them named rather than cured. It would surely be better to have them both named and cured. Then we hear of its being called peliosis, uric-acid-aemia or oxy-uri-chaemia, the very large number of names, barbarous and otherwise, showing the obscurity that attaches to the condition, both in the medical and the lay mind. The association of the disease with affection of the connective tissue and the consequent affixing to it of the name initis will help to dispel much of this obscurity and throw light on dark places.

XIX. SEQUENCES ON INITIS.

Diseases, mostly incurable, which follow on the long continued presence of initis in the body.

BEFORE going on to a detailed examination of the parts affected in initis and the treatment proper for them, let me just put before the reader again the steps of the processes by which its occurrence is connected with the general nutrition, and then look briefly at its serious consequences. First, then, we have dyspepia or mal-assimilation or indigestion; then we have connective-tissue congestion; and after that we have a long array of serious and often incurable affections, whose onset timely treatment might prevent or postpone often for years. The sequences in the various cases are the following, or the following are some of them, for the list is not complete:-

1. Dyspepsia, initis, inflammatory affections—as inflammation of the throat (tonsilitis), or colds—as bronchitis, pleurisy, broncho-pneumonia or pneumonia; or influenza with or without pneumonia; or the condition which is often termed "a severe feverish cold."

2. Dyspepsia, initis, recurrent or chronic bronchitis. This sequence occurs very frequently, and is quite easy to understand if we use the knowledge detailed in all books of anatomy to the effect that the breathing organs or lungs are formed as an outgrowth from the digestive tract. The lungs are therefore complementary digestive organs—that is to say, in plain English, we eat (and drink) the colds that we suffer from. All sufferers from recurring attacks of asthma and bronchitis, or at least almost all of them, are tender if pressed in the hollow of the breast-bone, and indeed are tender generally and wherever they are pressed; and often they are peliotic also. Attacks of bronchial or tracheal catarrh occur, and coincidently a connective—tissue congestion takes place in various situations, so that the two conditions are often simultaneous, though sometimes they are

successive also. If there is not complete recovery after each attack, as is often the case, then both of these conditions are slowly and intermittently aggravated, until in time some of the other consequences of dyspepsia and initis occur, as will be set forth immediately.

3. Dyspepsia, initis, tuberculosis.

4. Dyspepsia, initis, Bright's disease of the kidneys.

5. Dyspepsia, initis, apoplexy.

6. Dyspepsia, initis, meningitis—i.e. inflammation of the membranes of the brain or spinal cord, the patient dying with effusion, and perhaps comatose. A small proportion of so-called hysterical patients are carried off often this way, death occurring unexpectedly after three or four days.

7. Dyspepsia, initis, cancer.

8. Dyspepsia, initis, insanity. After a period of time, during which the patient develops flightiness of character and irregularity of mental action, insanity not infrequently supervenes, with or without general paralysis; or it may be with sclerosis of the spinal cord.

9. Dyspepsia, initis, angina pectoris. In my experience, angina pectoris, which is cramp of the heart, is always preceded or accompanied by *periostitis sterni*, or inflammation of the coverings of the breast-bone. And it is generally also accompanied by congestion of the fibrous bands which proceed from the back of the sternum or breast-bone to the pericardium. Cramp is over-contraction of muscular fibre, and when this cramp overtakes the transverse fibres of the heart, death occurs in "inhibition," as it is called, or over-action. If the over-action affects the longitudinal elements of the heart and vessels, the patient equally dies, but in collapse with a quickened, running and weakening pulse. It is curious to reflect that death occurs in over-action in each case; in the former, with over-action of the transverse elements; in the latter, with over-action

of the longitudinal. We do not realise how often it is that death occurs, not from diminished but from increased action, not from deficiency but from excess of action. In ordinary cramp the heart is empty after death. When death occurs from collapse the heart cavities are full of blood.

10. Dyspepsia, initis, peri-typhlitis or appendicitis. In many cases of peri-typhlitis the connective tissue around the caecum inflames and suppurates and an abscess forms, which either is opened by the surgeon or it may be opened by nature into the nearest intestinal coil, and so be emptied into the outer world.

In all these conditions, and in others not mentioned, the initic state is the intermediate one, indigestion or mal-assimilation or dyspepsia being the first. Like the embryonic development of animals which pass on almost indistinguishable from one another in early stages, however different they are going to become later, the development of these diseases passes through the two stages of dyspepsia or mal-assimilation and initis or connective-tissue congestion, before the characteristic signs of the later stages are developed. In the initial condition the symptoms are often those of depression of temperature and of the vital energies, including sometimes slowing of the pulse with languor and inanition—signs which are usually considered to indicate the need for increased feeding, whereas, the condition being usually one of blocking and congestion, the very reverse mode of management is generally indicated and ought to be recommended. But the main consideration to be kept in mind is, that, had the dyspepsia and initis been dealt with in time, and properly dealt with, they would have proved amenable to cure, and so the fatal diseases and consequences of these conditions would either have been prevented or would have been postponed for a time more or less long, or for a number of years.

Of course it will be evident to the reader that there is a philosophy underlying the considerations here advanced. And the prevailing philosophy (nearly always held even by those will sneer at it and think that they despise philosophy, although no human being can get on without it) is in complete and determined opposition to it. As long as we hold that the strength manifested through the body, and that the heat of the body depend on the food ingested into it, so long will the philosophical view that bodily energy and bodily heat depend on the force of life animating the body meet with fierce opposition. Obviously if bodily strength and heat or bodily temperature depend on food, then diminished heat and impaired strength must be met by increased amounts of food and not by restriction of it. But fires may be put out by heaping up too much coal on to them; and while lowered temperature may no doubt arise from taking too little food into the body, the temperature of the body may also be diminished by ingesting too much; and in fact this is far more frequently the cause of a too low bodily temperature than the other.

A great physician of the last generation, or of the last generation but one, frequently reminded his colleagues and his patients that there is a "starvation of over-repletion," and that many persons suffered from it. I cannot deal with this here, though it has been often dealt with before, nor do I wish to complicate the present considerations by arguing it. Suffice it that the reader is reminded that it exists, and that it is essential for him to make up his mind upon it, for his health and even his life depend upon the way in which he settles it. I believe that if we could get to understand this question properly, and if, understanding it, we allowed our conduct to be swayed by our views, we might be able to add a large number of years, fifteen or twenty or twenty-five or more, to healthy, happy and efficient human life. This is a very important consideration. To add even five years to the life of the forty-five millions of people living in the United Kingdom would mean the adding of two hundred and twenty-five millions of years of life to the present passing generation; while the addition of an average of twenty-five years would amount to the enormous total of five times that, or one thousand two hundred and twenty-five millions of years added to the lifetime of the same generation. What this addition to healthy human life might mean to the industrial, social, moral and spiritual life of the people is beyond human power to depict (especially as it would still be in our own option to use it for good and noble purposes or for bad or less noble) but it is surely of the greatest importance that we should make up our minds whether we think it is attainable or not. And the reader may perhaps be induced to reflect to what purposes might be put an addition of even five years to the average duration of life of the fifteen or sixteen hundred millions of human beings now living on the face of our globe. For these considerations, as they are general, affect all human beings alike, white, yellow, black or red.

XX. THE FREQUENCY OF THE OCCURRENCE OF CASES OF INITIS.

CASES of initis are very common. Hundreds, if not thousands, of them come under the notice of every practitioner of medicine, or might come under his notice if he chose to look for them. To describe such cases at length would therefore be to recount the details of ordinary medical practice. So common are they that in my case-books they are entered simply as cases of *morbus vulgaris,* or the common disease; and sometimes the word *peliosis* is added when this frequently concomitant condition is also present. Common, however, as they are, some cases stand out in my memory, and among them one to which I venture to refer, because the young lady had been for years under the care of a competent, well qualified and experienced practitioner, with little or no improvement in her condition, and got well in a few months when proper or, let us say, different treatment was adopted. The patient was a religeuse in a convent and was thirty years of age. Another religeuse, a trained nurse, wrote me letters respecting the patient before I saw her. She said that the patient had been in the convent for four years.

"During the first two years" (the nurse said), "she had what appeared to be bilious, attacks, recurring about every two months. These sometimes lasted two or three days or a week. She never actually vomited, but felt very sick. The colour of her face was a greenish yellow, but the eyes were not tinged. The doctor saw her, and he sent her medicine for the liver, which did not seem to be of much benefit to her. The third year the attacks became more frequent, coming on about every month. In January 1909 she looked very ill, and complained of pain in the left side of the abdomen. She also had leucorrhoeal discharge. The doctor was called again, and I asked him to make a thorough examination, which he did. He said the liver was perfectly sound, but the uterus was a little prolapsed, and there was some inflammation in the ovaries, which would account for the pain." (Congestion of connective tissue in the abdomen—abdominal initis ?—A.R.) "I told him of her constipated state and that she was obliged to take aperients almost every night. He ordered treatment for the abdominal pain. She was also to take a pill at night and to have an enema in the morning. This treatment was to be continued for a few weeks."

The letter then goes on to describe how blocked the bowels were, and when the attending doctor heard of this

"he said the bowels were ulcerated, and that the patient was suffering from foecal poisoning. In about four weeks she seemed to rally, and the doctor discontinued his visits. For a week or so she kept fairly well, and then the old pain and feeling of sickness returned, and from time to time the attacks came on about every ten days." (The cause continuing, the attacks are periodic or intermittent; and the longer the causes continue and increase, the shorter will be the intervals between the attacks; till by and by the attacks will never pass off completely, and the case will become chronic.—A.R.) "While the attack lasts, she is not able to take her food, and complains of rather severe pain and sickness just before and after the bowels act."

So the narrative goes on, and it is added, "the doctor seems to think the patient is suffering from hysteria." The patient was then, at the request of the convent superior, taken into a private ward at a hospital and remained there for a fortnight, during which time she was treated mostly by injections and purgatives—but without improvement. I saw the patient in the month of July, and in three months dismissed her cured. I recommended the application of hot linseed meal poultices to the abdomen every night for an hour for six weeks, and restricted the diet from four to two meals a day, and recommended general exercises for five minutes in the act of dressing in the morning. By and by the exercises were to be continued for ten minutes, and later for fifteen minutes; but they were never to be continued for longer than this. Under this treatment the patient recovered her vigour and much of her colour; the greeny-yellow colour disappeared; she got rid of her inveterate constipation without taking aperients, and also got rid of her other symptoms.

To the very good clinical account of the case written by a trained nurse, I add that when I saw the patient, she was pale and languid looking, and I found, on examining her, the signs and symptoms of what I regard as general initis or congestion of the connective tissues all over the body. She was tender at the back of the neck, in the ligaments that attach the head to the neck, and in the muscles of the back and sides of the neck. The joints of the jaws were also tender, and so were the muscles of the cheeks and jaws. So were the supra-orbital and infra-orbital nerve sheaths. In a like condition also were the erector spinae muscles or muscles of the back, causing the pain between the shoulders, of which men and women in this condition so often complain, and of which this patient complained. There was also tenderness of the sternum or breast-bone (*periosiitis sterni*) premonitory of the later onset of *angina pectoris*, although it would probably have been many years before this ensued. There was also tenderness of the articulations between the ribs and the breast-bone, a true arthritis or inflammation of the joints, no doubt. The young woman was also tender in a great many other places in the body—in fact, in all the places shown in the illustrations to this book. It would not be inappropriate to say that she suffered from rheumatic neuralgia or myalgia, or myalgic or neuralgic rheumatism all over the body more or less. Not only was the front of the breast-bone tender, but I have no doubt that the back of it (had we been able to reach it) would have been found tender to pressure also, and that there was congestion of the sterno-pericardial bands which pass from the back of the breast-bone to the pericardium. When a long-continued congestion creeps along these bands, inflammation is often conveyed to the pericardium, and to the heart itself, and, in this insidious way, slowly arising heart disease often sets in. At least these are the steps of the changes slowly occurring, which appear not infrequently to lead at a later stage of the illness, to the occurrence of *angina pectoris*, and to sudden death with rheumatic cramp of the heart.

In the case in question the important consideration is that a diagnosis of general initis followed by appropriate treatment cured the patient, who had suffered for years. The dyspeptic nature of the ailment accounts for the recurring bilious attacks which were due to congestion of gall-bladder, stomach and duodenum; for the abdominal pain which was due to connective tissue congestion of the lower abdomen; for the inveterate constipation which was no doubt accompanied by connective-tissue congestion of the intestine itself; and for the general languor, pallor and feeling of malaise which prevented her from attending to her duties, as well as for the suggestion of "hysteria" which is often such an aggravation of the sufferings of sensitive women apt to be driven to despair by their conviction that no one understands their ailments and that the science and art of medicine are powerless to suggest means of relief.

That there is no proof in the scientific sense of the existence of the initis which is in my opinion nearly always present in these affections, that no microscopic examination of the affected tissues was made, or of the tissues alleged to be affected, leaves me entirely unmoved. Would a medical man be justified in asking leave to cut down on the back of the neck or over the gall bladder or down to the Fallopian tubes, in order to remove a portion of the tissues and to submit it to microscopic examination? The suggestion is barbarous and ridiculous and unnecessary. The evidence for the existence of the condition is probable evidence no doubt, and it is moral evidence and it is clinical; but it is evidence of the same kind as serves for the general conduct of life; and I am as sure of its cogency as if a hundred microscopical examinations and painful demonstrations had certified it or had failed to demonstrate what in the early stages is probably too fugitive to be demonstrable, although it is not too fugitive to cause great annoyance to the patient. Clinical and probable and moral evidence led to the formation of the diagnosis, and treatment in accordance with the diagnosis led to the cure of the patient. Some day perhaps there may be micro-scopic corroborative evidence—or it may be impossible to produce it. If the former, we shall be grateful for more light. But if the latter, I do not think we ought to cease trying to cure our patients because we are still short of some corroborative evidence as to their condition. It seems true that the limits of experimental inquiry are very soon reached when we are dealing with vital phenomena, even although the limits between the phenomena of the living and the not-living (if there are any not-living phenomena) are very difficult or even impossible to define.

A word or two may be said here as to the constipation of the bowels which accompanied the general affection. This was due to over-contraction of the transverse muscular fibres of the intestine and was caused by over-nutrition. When the daily meals were reduced from four to two, it disappeared. Constipation is the commonest condition in these states and is as common among men as among women, being due to the same cause in both sexes. Sometimes, however, diarrhoea occurs, and is due to over-stimulation and to over-contraction of the longitudinal elements of the intestine. The bowel being a tube whose walls are constructed mainly of two sets of elements, one transverse or circular and passing across its width, and the other longitudinal or passing along its length (like the weft and warp of a cloth) over-stimulation and over-contraction of either of these may occur. If over-contraction of the transverse elements occurs, obviously the tube will be narrowed and lengthened, and it will be difficult for the contents to pass along, because resistance will be offered to their passage. This condition will translate itself into constipation. If, on the other hand, over-stimulation of the longitudinal elements occur, the bowel-tube will be shortened and widened, and the contents will be hurried through, and of course in this case diarrhoea will appear. And this also explains how the same treatment will be called for in the management of both constipation and diarrhoea, because the indication is to remove the over-stimulation in both cases, in the one case the over-stimulation and over-contraction of the transverse elements, and in the other the over-stimulation and over-contraction of the longitudinal. The over-stimulation being in both cases due to over-nutrition, diminution of food is indicated in both conditions. And so a restriction of the meals from four or five to two a day, even if their quality is not altered, will cure both constipation on the one hand, and diarrhoea on the other. And if, as sometimes happens, the patient suffers at one time from constipation, and at another from diarrhoea, both of these alternating conditions will be cured by the same treatment.

These are not merely theoretical considerations; they are very practical also, for I have been able in many cases by applying them, to cure both constipation and diarrhoea, as also the alternation of the one state on the other—that is, I have been able so to advise patients as that they have been enabled to cure themselves. Doctors, it is true, cure nothing. It is the force of life that cures, by altering the body so as to render it fit for the habitation of life. But doctors may often advise patients to act so that the force of life may have free course, and so have or make the opportunity of curing them. The force of life, human-animal-life, or equine or canine or vulpine or elephantine, pithecoid or other, procreates the body of the animal, rendering it {it for its own habitation originally, and then tends to keep it fit for that purpose afterwards; and so when it is out of order, to restore it to the order of health. That this is all done unconsciously only deepens my sense of the guidance and direction under which the life-force unconsciously works towards health and harmony, and suggests the anticipation of the time when what it now does unconsciously it may then do consciously, making for itself a mechanism fit for this end. Of the two views (a) that the life is the effect of the organisation of the body, and (b) that the life makes the body to be a place fit for its habitation, the second seems far the more likely, for it is far more probable that the life is the cause of the body, than that the body is the cause of the life. This is how the case stands if we are compelled to choose between these two opposite and contending views. But, as was shown before, we are not compelled to make this choice, since a fuller and no doubt the more correct View is that the body and the life inhabiting it or manifested in it are not cause and effect of one another, but are on the other hand, concomitant effects of a common cause—viz. the universal omnipotent and eternal energy whereby all things do consist, and which continually emanates from the only source adequate to account for it.

These considerations, however, explain the paradox that the same causes acting on the organism (over-stimulation and over-contraction, in the instances before us) often induce states so opposite as constipation and diarrhoea, and help to explain the general paradox that the same causes often induce opposite states, and how the same treatment is indicated for the cure of both. And the other paradox that frequently occurs in medicine (and in life also, for that matter, for practical medicine deals with one set of the conditions of life)—viz. that opposite causes often induce the same or similar states becomes intelligible also. For a little study enables us to understand how the effects of too much are often apparently the same as the effects of too little, and how there may be a starvation of over-repletion as well as a starvation of under-feeding.

The medical adviser may be justified, nay, he may even be compelled to advise restriction of the diet in the case of the thin, the attenuated and the wasted as well as in the over-grown and the obese, though it is this practical application of his views which is so often a stumbling block to his clients.

In commercial life, business may be brought to a standstill in two opposite conditions—viz. (a) when stocks give out and (b) when stocks are too heavy. In the former state business ceases because there are no stocks to buy or sell; but in the latter business is choked and hindered because, the stocks being too heavy and the market being glutted, the merchant is afraid to buy or sell, since he is afraid that, instead of making a profit, he may sustain a loss.

Whatever may be the ease in commercial life, and whatever may be the chief cause of stagnation in the body commercial, in the body physical, inanition and attenuation are far oftener caused by the ingestion of too much than by the ingestion of too little.

PART II.
SYSTEMATIC AND REPEATED EXERCISES.

THE performance of systematic movements offers the advantage of stimulating, if unconsciously, all the functions which we have seen to be subserved by the connective tissue, the functions of conductivity of impressions, of common response and common sensibility, the feeling of general well-being and of the unity and solidarity of the body. Repeated and systematic exercises also bring into use the action of muscles which the business of life does not call upon, since that business usually consists of the repetition of the same muscular actions over and over and over again, while that of others is omitted and neglected through disuse. It will be well therefore to consider and depict muscular actions in systematic order. This order is no doubt more or less arbitrary, and may be altered at the option of the person concerned or of the adviser. In point of fact, I often recommend commencing with the use of the exercise numbered 14 in the series, in order to emphasise the view that the connective tissues about the stomach and digestive organs generally ought to be relieved of their passive congestion first, and in order that we may always keep in mind the relation between the functions of digestion, assimilation and nutrition on the one hand and those of movement and work on the other. In truth, however, so long as the movements are performed, it does not matter very much in what order we take them; and so I am commencing with movements of the lower extremities.

In Figure 1 the person or patient (for often enough he is one without knowing it) is shown sitting on a chair, say, after the underclothing has been put on after the morning bath. If women wear corsets, it is better that they should not have them on. The person's thumbs are shown pressing against the inner edge of the tibia or shin-bone or leg-bone, where not infrequently it. is found to be tender on examination. The right knee is shown bent at a right angle, and the left ankle is laid by its outside on the bent knee. The knee of the limb which is laid on the other (in this case the left) ought to be well lowered, somewhat more even than is shown in the illustration, and then the thumbs should be passed, with pressure, along the edge of the shin-bone, until the upper thumb working from above down, gradually approaches the lower one, working from the ankle upwards. In this way the whole of the inner edge of the bone with its over-lying covering or periosteum can be manipulated, what tenderness there is can be manifested and gradually removed, and the blood circulation and the lymph circulation can both be stimulated. A considerable number, say twenty-five to thirty, or more, pressure movements should be effected by the thumbs on the bone. And then the exercise should be reversed, the left knee being bent and the right ankle laid on it, and treated in a similar way.

If the corresponding photograph had been taken, Figure 1 would have appeared as an *a* and *b* form, as is shown in the next figure. Tapping or hammering the whole flat surface of the shinbone with the fingers ought to be easily borne without pain; and I generally advise that a couple of hundreds of such taps be applied. If the parts are so tender that the tapping is badly borne, then we may infer that the periosteal connective tissue covering the bone is congested, and that we ought to pursue daily a course of treatment by movement,

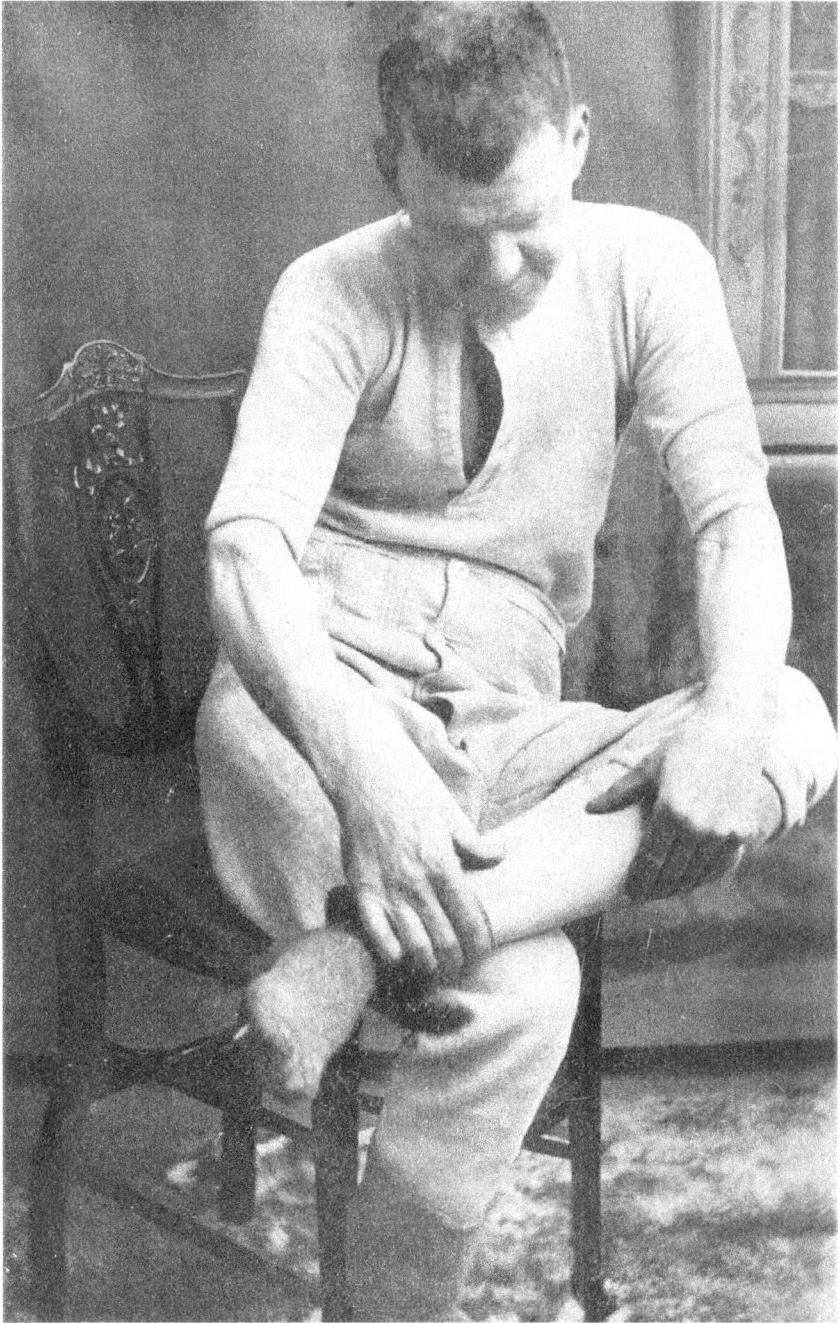

FIG. 1
Manipulation of the Shin bone.

pressure and tapping, alternated with short rests, until we get rid of it.

Movements should be instituted after the morning bath or in the act of dressing in the morning, and before any food is taken. This is the best time of the day for the movements, and the larger number of pressure movements should be effected then; but it is well to do, say, half or one-third of the number again before the last meal of the day. A good time is when the dress is changed for dinner or for evening, or before tea-time for working people.

Well-to-do people may perhaps in course of time come to learn the unwholesomeness and damage to health that arise from interpolating a meal at afternoon-tea time between lunch and dinner, since it is not required for nutrition at all; and can only serve to congest the connective tissues of the body. So far from doing any good, it thus does positive harm, since the blood, finding itself loaded with food-material beyond its requirements for the nutrition of the tissues, quickly and quietly drops the surplus into the connective tissues, there to be dealt with by the lymphatic system in the way already described. This system has been unconsciously introduced for scavengering purposes by the force of life, and yet with uses so economic that we might almost say that it was knowingly determined that nothing should be lost, since the lymphatics convey unused nutritive material back again into the blood for re-use. But when these unexpressed and unconscious designs are systematically and repeatedly opposed by the interpolation of too many meals or by taking too heavy meals, the circulation is apt to find itself blocked more and more, some time after each meal, and even after the elimination of waste which takes place during sleep; and so the person feels himself or herself tireder and tireder, more and more fatigued, heavy, dull, weak and run-down. The cup of tea taken alone, especially if weak, does not seem to me to be accompanied by these disadvantages, and seems to do good instead of harm. It seems to act as a stimulus to the stomach to complete the digestion of the previous meal, and its cheering effects are more perceptible than if it is taken along with the bread and butter and cakes or (sad to relate) the jam or marmalade sandwiches which, by a subtle perversion of taste and of nutrition, one sees sometimes eaten at such times. No wonder that the next clever doctor is compelled to recommend a course of treatment at Carlsbad or Harrogate in order that the wholesome waters may wash out. The waste matters which ought never to have been allowed to accumulate in the system. Perhaps even the exercises might have been unnecessary if this slow insidious loading and choking and blocking of the body had not been allowed to occur. And this is the reason, no doubt, why some medical authorities (notably Erasistratus, who lived about 300 B.C.) have said that exercises were not necessary for the health of the body. Until we learn better the meaning of nutrition, however, let us perform our exercises. But if, after return from Carlsbad or Harrogate, the same or similar habits are resumed—what then?

Let us draw a kindly and concealing veil over our delicacy, our subtlety, our refinement. We are delicate, no doubt, but how did we become so? And if pursuing certain habits has made us so, and if an alteration in our way of living has for the time being improved our health, will not a return to our former habits be likely to make us ill again? In parts of the body like the shin-bone we are sometimes, or indeed often, both numb and tender at the same time. We do not feel pressure or contact sufficiently if it is slight, a mere touch, for instance; and on the other hand, we feel it too much and too painfully, if an appreciable amount of pressure is exerted on the part. This paradox of feeling too much and too little through the same tissues at the same time seems to be explained if we remember that, theoretically, animal structures are made up of two sets of fibres, one, the transverse, whose contraction narrows and lengthens parts. If this contraction of the transverse fibres is pushed further into over-action, the over-action translates itself into numbness, and if it is pushed further still, cramp is experienced like that felt by the swimmer; or sea-bather who loses his life through the onset of cramp or over-contraction in his muscles. Contraction or action of the other set of fibres, the longitudinal, causes shortening and widening of parts; and if the action is still more stimulated, tenderness and pain ensue, followed, if the action is further persisted in, by collapse. This over-action has been termed inhibition because normal physiological action is prevented or inhibited, and a new set of facts appears. Contraction of the transverse elements causes defect or lowering of function, or at least is accompanied by this physiological state, the end being cramp and numbness. Contraction of the longitudinal fibres, by causing shortening and widening, is accompanied by heightening of function, the end or termination being tenderness and collapse.

Death which leads to the cessation of life or which may be said to be the cessation of one form of life, thus usually occurs from excess of action and not from the defect of action or from the inanition, which, we generally think, accompanies it. Occasionally death does seem to occur from inanition or failure of function, and not from excess of function; but this form or mode of death occurs far less frequently than it ought to do. We may also notice how loosely and vaguely we talk about death, since, when the human force of life leaves the human body, or when the horse-life-force or the elephant-life-force leave the body of a horse or an elephant, these bodies are by no means dead, but become immediately the seat of lower forms of life, which, in plant or animal form, consume the body from which the higher form of life has departed. The forms of life which inhabit the body of a man, a horse, or an elephant might be termed respectively anthropino-zoo-dynamic, hippo-zoo-dynamic, and elephanto-zoo-dynamic. They are, each of them, varieties of the one universal energy whereby all things do consist. A little extension indeed of this reasoning soon shows us or induces us to believe that the whole universe is alive with energy which moves and lives in higher and lower and lowest forms known under the names of various forces, as electro-dynamic, chemico-dynamic, and crystallo-dynamic, down to hydro-dynamic and hylo-dynamic or gravitation, and through all pervading aethereo-dynamic.

Life and death come to be, when analysed, not contradictories, the one excluding its contradictory for ever; but contraries only in the sense of being manifestations of higher or lower forms of life. Not life and death then form our experience, but more life or less life, the differences being not of kinds but of degrees only. In this sense there is no death. Everything is the incarnation of some form or phase or variety of the universal energy whereby all things do consist. And only if the infinite eternal and omnipotent source of this energy were to cease to be—only then would or could the universe be empty of the life with which it now abounds in all degrees, from what we call (but foolishly and illogically) inanimate forms to plant and animal forms which we call animate—only then could any parts of the universe be dead. More animate or less animate, not animate and inanimate, is the universe which we experience.

The qualities of infinity, omnipotence and eternity by no means exhaust the characteristics of the universal energy, for we have to attribute to it wisdom, design, mercy, love, and other characteristics with which it is not the province of this present writing to deal, although the principles which dictate the written words must, if true, be found to be in harmony with those that manifest themselves in other departments of the universe in which we live. The presence of numbness and tenderness at the same time in the same part, the paradox by which a tissue is the instrument of defect of function and of excess of function at the same time, is thus found to be exceedingly interesting as raising issues which we had not realised as being connected with it.

If we properly understood nutrition, and if, understanding it, we attempted to carry our understanding into the practical government of the body, neither the numbness nor the tenderness would exist, and the human body would remain the normal habitation of anthropino—zoo—dynamic for a very much longer time than it does now. We too often attribute to our ancestors obscure ailments which are mostly of our own bringing on. If our ancestors suffered from them, whence did they get them? From their ancestors in turn? Questions like these are apt sometimes to make us imagine or declare that it is neither we nor our ancestors but Fate that is to blame for the evils from which we suffer. But this is a short-sighted conclusion. Ailments, if not universal, probably began at some time in human history, and probably also recur in successive generations, as similar causes affect the bodies of similarly constituted men. Successive generations of weary Willies and tired Tims and Sarah Janes that have always to be lying down, have to be accounted for. And we have also to consider whether work-cures or rest-cures are most suitable for them. Probably the advice that they should do less digestive work and more useful work, that they should labour their organisms less with tropho-dynamic and more with erg-dynamic would be better for them, if it might not be so palatable. But the body is fitted to be the instrument not only of erg-dynamic but also of noetico-dynamic, and of aesthetico-dynamic and of even higher forms of work; and if such heavy digestive labour as we generally subject it to were not indulged in, there would be more scope and power for thinking, feeling, and the exercise of higher emotions and qualities still.

If only we could free ourselves of the double delusion that the force manifested through the body and the heat of the body was dependent on the food, there might be some hope of our understanding the proper function of nutrition-viz. the restoration of the waste incurred in the adult body by the action of the force of life that inhabits it. Perhaps I should not say a double but a treble delusion, for we have been recently authoritatively told that scientific men do not admit the existence of a force of life. It does not seem to be recognised that to determine this question demands the use of philosophy, and that the eminence of men or their pre-eminence in science is no necessary passport to their philosophical attainment. It might be well to inquire perhaps whether the assumption of the existence of infinite, omnipotent, and eternal energy constantly made by scientific men involves the admission of the existence of life-force, for it is possible that this universal energy is itself alive, and that it is constantly translating itself into or incarnating itself in what we call living things on the one hand, and into what we call not living on the other. The view that the life-force is a variety of the universal energy would, it seems to me, much simplify this discussion, and would make many obscure things plainer than they are. A living energy will not be likely to make a dead universe. Meantime, let us gratefully accept and thankfully use the discoveries of science, and let us call upon our reason and judgment for our philosophy. A proper understanding of the function of nutrition, with the attempt to exercise the proper restraint which nature inculcates in all directions, even if it made us exclaim—who is sufficient for these things?—would result not in less but in greater efficiency of our bodies as the instruments of work, while it would result also in a great increase in the duration of what we call life, as also in a great diminution of the illnesses incident to it.

In Figure 2, *a* and *b*, a similar position of the limb is shown; but the thumbs are now manipulating the muscles of the calf (the gastrocnemius and soleus as they are called) rather than the periosteum of the shin bone. The foot of the laid-on limb is moved forward and backward, or flexed (*a*) and extended (*b*), as the movements are termed. In effecting the pressure while the movements are being performed, the person will discover how very tender the muscles of the calf are, and how painful on pressure and movement are the coverings of the muscles (the perimysium), and he or she will probably be astonished at the amount of tenderness elicited. Movements as shown, and repeated daily, or twice daily, are highly efficacious in enabling us to get rid of the tenderness; and this translates itself into a lightness and ease of movement, as in walking or running, which require to be felt in order to be appreciated.

In doing these movements the first effect no doubt often is to aggravate the tenderness, and may even be to make it rise from dull aching into pain. If the pain is very severe, we should desist from the movements for a day, or even two days; but we should not give them up, for the putting of the parts into use or action is essential if they are ever to become the efficient instruments of the body and its indwelling life-force. Efficiency can be effected only through use and not through inactivity, or rather, through use, followed at short intervals by periods of inactivity—that is, by motion followed by rest; and this general statement must be understood as being true of all bodily movements whatever. In the

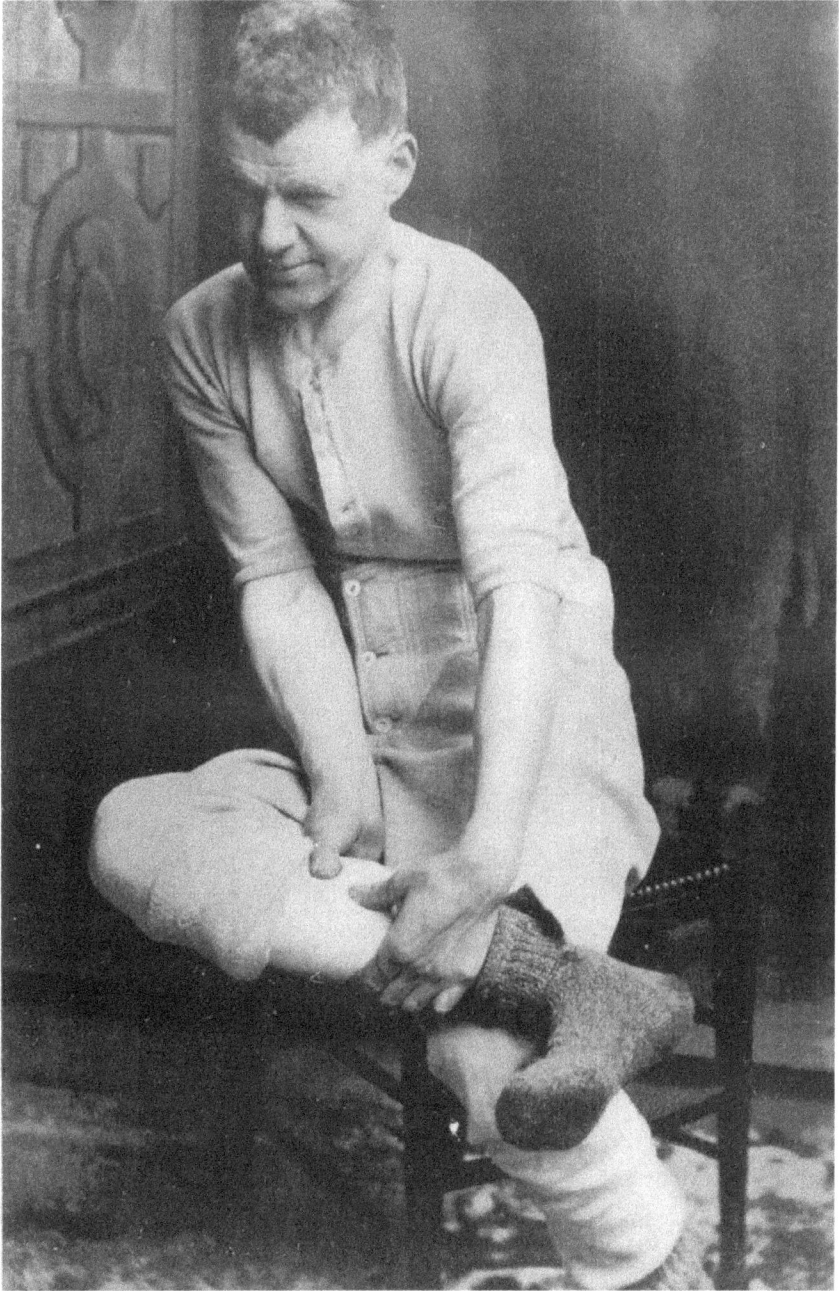

FIG. 2a

Manipulation of the Calf of the Leg and also of the Muscles of the Front
of the Leg.

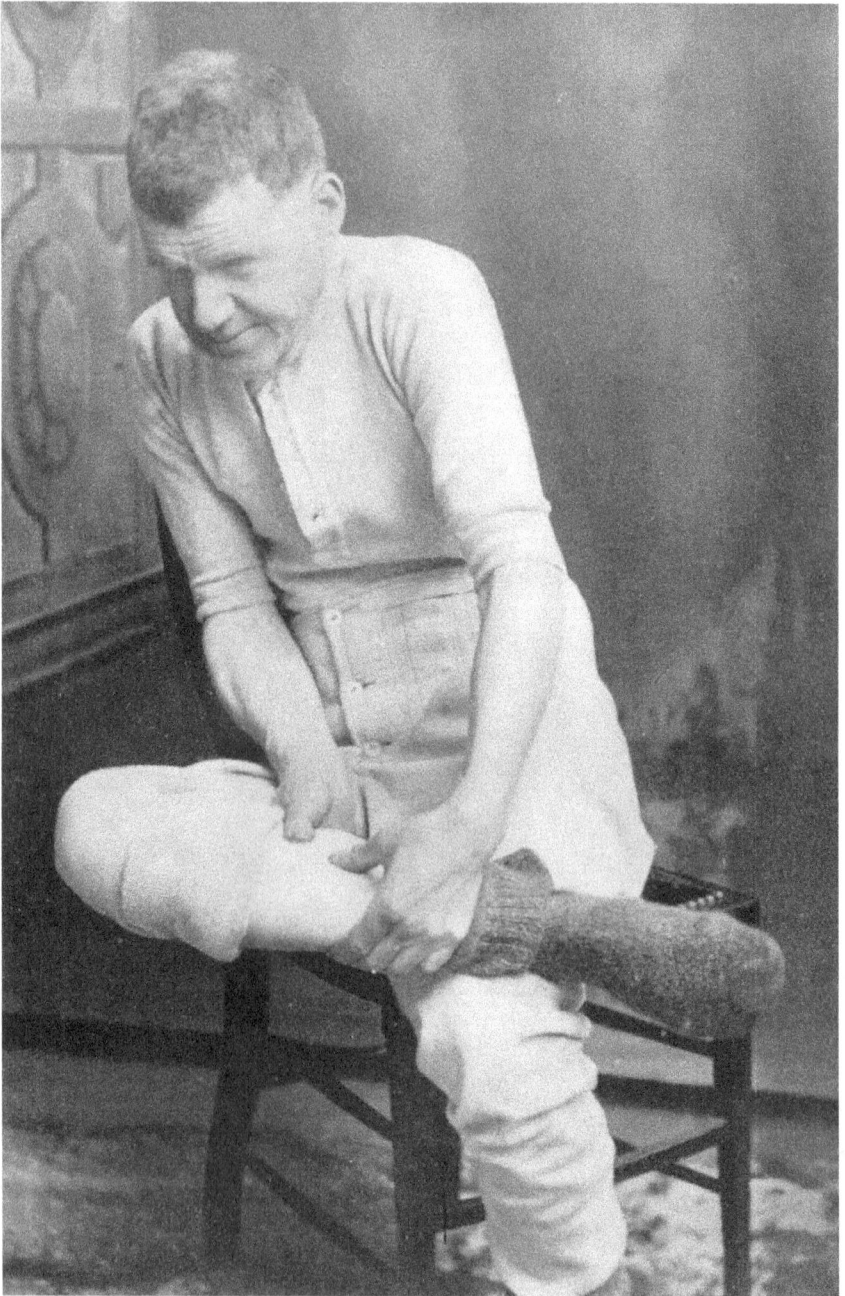

FIG. 2b

Manipulation of the Calf of the Leg and also of the Muscles of the Front of the Leg.

prosecution of the business of life, many movements are unused or discontinued altogether, but this is not wise. The body is apt to lose the power or to forget how to do movements which it is not being constantly called upon to do, and this is the chief reason why the performance of general movements daily is so desirable. Of course, persons need not confine the movements to the precise points shown in the photographs. Much benefit will be got by free manipulation of all the muscles and of their surrounding connective tissues; and it is hoped that pressure movements will be gradually extended to all parts of the limbs, so as to dissipate the congestion and tenderness which weigh them down. This observation, like the other, is also a general observation, and extends to all movements of the body.

In Figure 3 (overleaf), manipulation of the foot is shown. The points shown are the joint between the first metatarsal bone (which carries the great toe) and the internal cuneiform, under the performer's or the masseur's thumb. The middle finger of the operator is shown pressing against the joint between the fifth metatarsal bone (carrying the small toe) and the cuboid bone, as it is called, on the outside of the foot. The thumb and fingers are pressed against the joints while the foot is being moved. As in other parts, pressure movements should be extended to all parts of the foot, when persons will be surprised to find how many points are tender to pressure. A place often found to be so is when pressure is made between the great toe and the one next to it. Pressure exerted between the other toes frequently compels us to draw the same conclusion and fills us with the same surprise. The slow silting up of the connective-tissue is in fact insidiously going on in the persons of the vast majority of us, if not in all of us without exception, although so few of us suspect it; and indeed after it has been pointed out, comparatively few of us are willing to undertake the trouble to attempt to get rid of it.

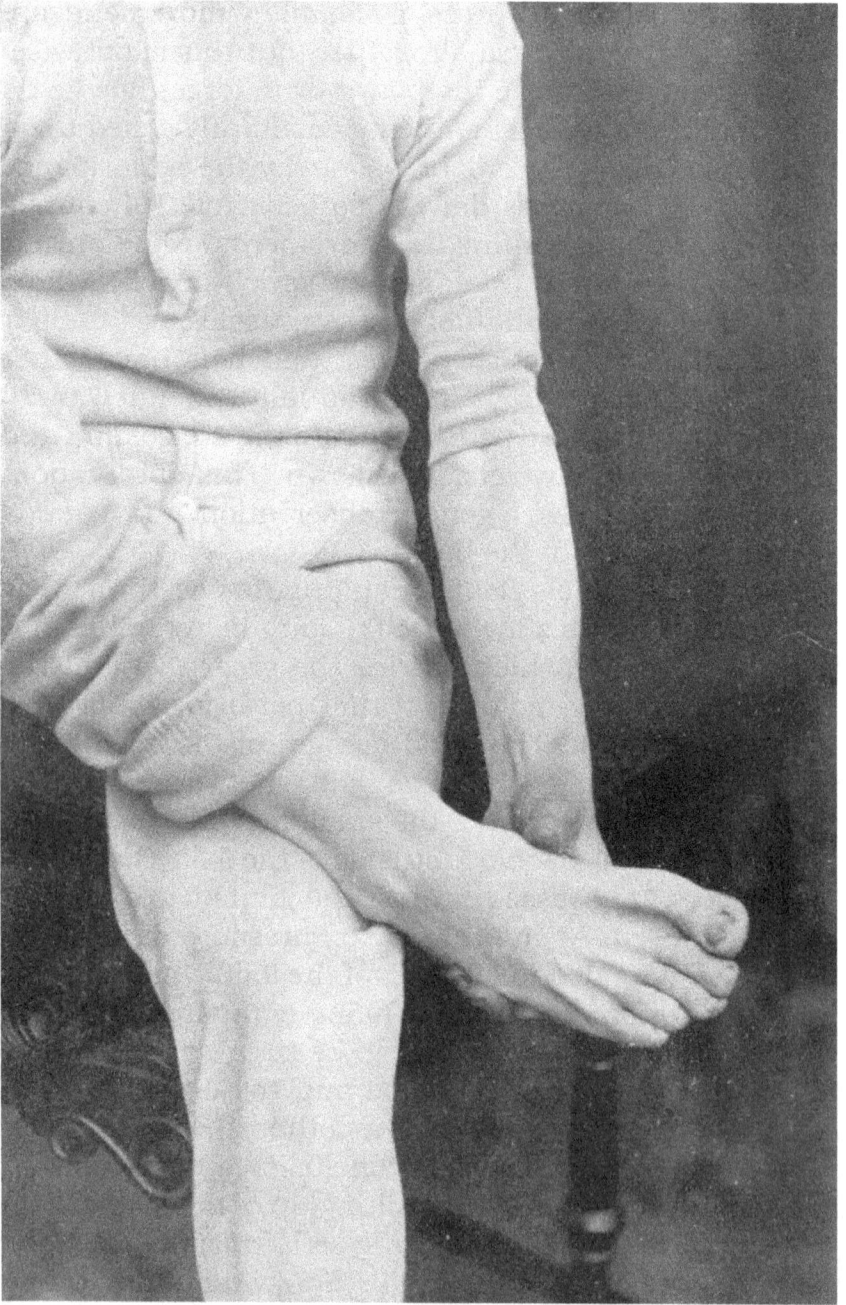

FIG. 3
Manipulation of the Foot.

An excellent way of manipulating the feet under pressure is to use the weight of the body itself for the purpose. This can be done by the simple means of rising on the balls of the toes and then coming back on to the soles of the feet and on to the heels. This movement, effected twenty-five or thirty times, has an admirable effect in freeing the movements of the feet and in enabling us to walk better and more freely. As in other cases, if we find it difficult to do twenty-five or thirty movements, we can begin with a dozen, or even fewer. We need not over-fatigue ourselves with doing too many movements at first. If a dozen movements are too many, we can do six or eight. It is well to begin with fewer movements, and to go on to more afterwards, than to weary ourselves at the beginning and then to imagine that the treatment does not suit us. It is necessary to persevere if we wish to be well; and even to persevere intermittently at repeated times and not to do too much at once. Conditions which have set in in the body insidiously and a long time ago cannot be expected to disappear at once, or even very soon. A patient who is recommended to take medicine three times a day would be very unwise to proceed to take a whole bottleful at once; and so it is with the effects of exercises which must be prosecuted at intervals, and not too continuously until the body is over-fatigued by them. Generally speaking, a ten minutes' use of them in the morning and for half of that time in the afternoon affords as much exercise as the body requires or will benefit by. At the very most, fifteen minutes is the longest time that need ever be spent at these movements; and five or six minutes, or possibly ten, in the afternoon. These may seem short periods of time in view of the hours that are spent on golf-courses and in motoring, cycling, etc., not to mention other games at the present time. Persons who have leisure will of course use it as they think proper. It is possible to make amusement the main business of life, and each man's taste and judgment and conscience must determine his conduct.

I am considering here what is necessary or at least highly desirable for the man and woman who wish to devote their lives to work, of whatever sort it may be. And those even I think who do mechanical work are better for the use of movements of this sort once or twice a day, since the business of life, even when it consists of doing mechanical work, implies the frequent repetition of some movements (perhaps a good many) but also involves the neglect of others. I have seen and been surprised at the existence of general initis in all sorts of persons, those whose business was the doing of mechanical work not excepted, and so I think it well to recommend these movements to all persons, whatever be their occupations; although no doubt they are more strongly indicated for persons doing the ordinary work of life, professional people, business people, clerks, literary people, housekeepers, etc., than perhaps for people doing mechanical work. And to do them twice a day seems to me to be better than only once, because the organism appears to forget, as it were, the effects of the morning lesson, if it is not repeated till next day. Even so, it is not wise to begin with fifteen minutes, it being much better to do so with five or six, and for half of that time in the afternoon. We can continue after this fashion for a week or so before increasing the number of the movements. Delicate women who bruise easily will also be well advised to use the movements very gently, so that by becoming gradually accustomed to them, their tissues may become firmer and harder and more elastic; and afterwards a little more vigour of motion may be allowed, and the use of movements for a longer time. But in no case is it necessary to spend a very long time over the movements.

Figure 4 *a* and *b* (overleaf). In this figure the person is again represented sitting. He is pressing with the fingers of the two hands firmly against the heads of the two bones of the leg, the tibia or shin-bone on the inner side, and the fibula on the outer side of the limb. At the same time he bends or flexes the leg as shown in 4*b* and again straightens or extends it as shown in 4*a*. The operator's middle finger is pressing against a point just below the knee-joint on the inner side which is often found to be tender. It is here that the sartorius muscle is inserted, and the strands of connective tissue by which it is attached to the tibia or shin-bone are often surprisingly tender. Not infrequently this tenderness is premonitory of trouble which may spread to the knee-joint itself at some subsequent time. This shows the importance of dealing with the affection in its early stages.

The sartorius is a very long muscle, extending from the anterior superior spine of the ilium right up at the top of the thigh on the outside down to its insertion at the inside of the upper part of the tibia or shin-bone. The action of the muscle is to raise the extended leg and thigh and to lift it a little laterally, and it can be well seen going into contraction when this movement is effected. The muscle can then be seen crossing the thigh in its whole length obliquely from the outer to the inner side, small at the top, and bigger and fleshier below. It is not infrequently tender all along its course to this position, but it ought not to be so if persons lived properly as regards food and movements. The insertion of the sartorius muscle is inseparably blended with the strands by which the inner ham-string muscles (the semi-membranous and semi-tendinosus as they are called) are inserted. They can be easily felt if we examine the inner side of the back of the knee while we move the leg. So true is it that all the connective tissues are all united or connected to one another.

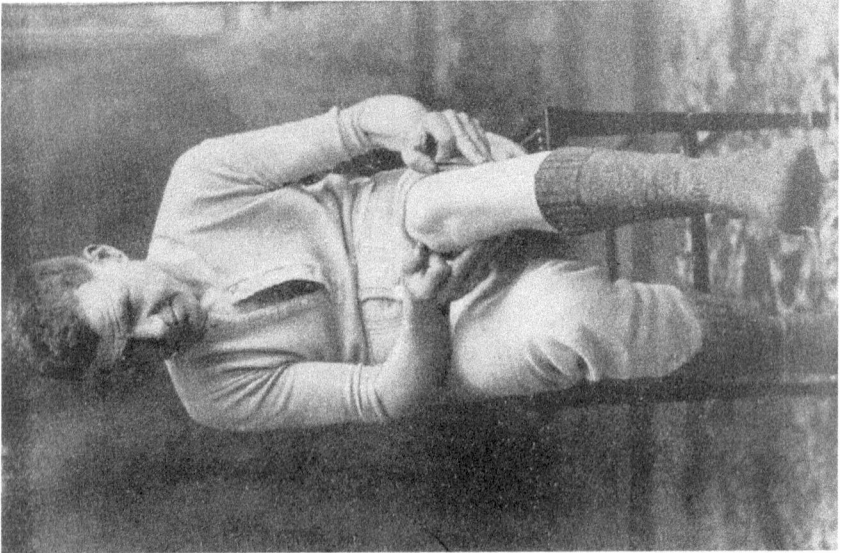

FIG. 4a

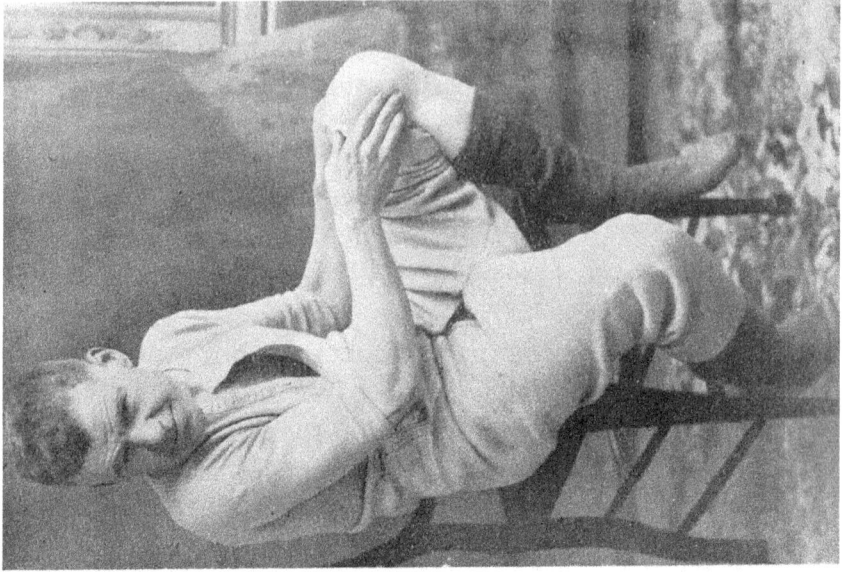

FIG. 4b

Pressure movements of the Knee-joint.

110

Figure 5*a* and 5*b* (overleaf) shows a valuable movement of the muscles of the thighs. The young woman is shown pressing firmly with the lingers into the inner and outer sides of what are known as the quadriceps extensor muscles of the thighs, as she bends down into the sitting position and rises again into the erect one. These muscles often ache obscurely, and the aching makes their owner feel tired when she begins to walk or do any work, and often indeed before she begins to walk or work. This was the condition existing in the case of the young nun formerly referred to, the connective tissues covering the muscles of the body being in a state of obscure indefinite unlocalised congestion and ache. This was also the condition in the young woman from whom the photograph was taken. Both of them got well.

In these situations of the body, peliosis is not infrequently found, the blacking and blueing being due to excessive friability and rupture of the connective tissues covering these muscles. The strands are so weak that they tear easily on the slightest exertion, or sometimes apparently with no exertion at all, and as they are torn, so are also the finest capillary blood-vessels and lymph-vessels which accompany them. The torn vessels bleed under the skin, showing the familiar discolorations. A similar state of nutrition of the parts surrounding the blood-vessels inside the head and the weakness accompanying it, leads to rupture of vessels there—that is, to apoplexy. It is through reflecting on considerations of this sort that we come to comprehend the urgent need that there is of dealing with this sort of affection before serious damage has yet been done by it in vital parts of the body. Or one should rather say- how important it is to see the causes of the evils that are occurring in the body, with a view to obviating them, and so, if possible, of preventing the occurrence in vital parts of conditions which are annoying and serious enough in

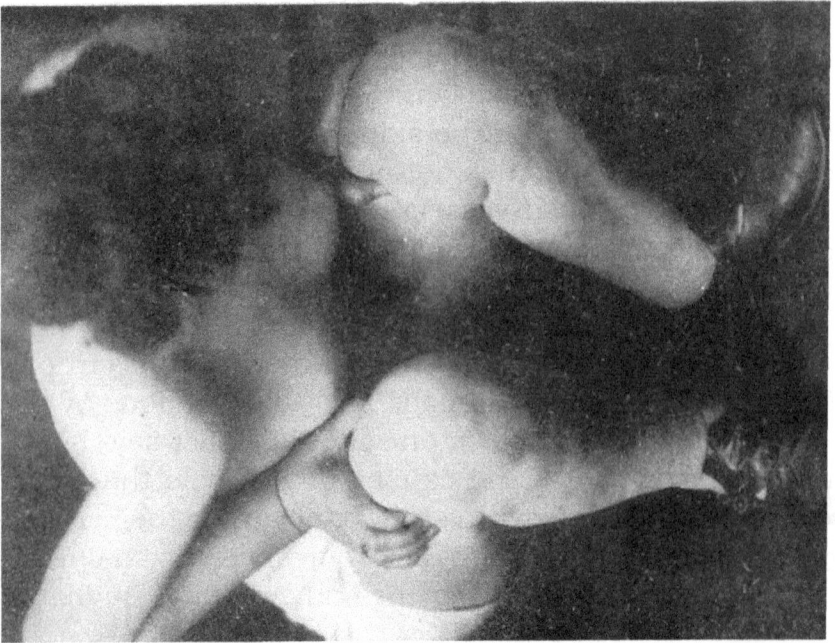

FIG. 5a

FIG. 5b

Self-movements under pressure of the Muscles of the Thighs.

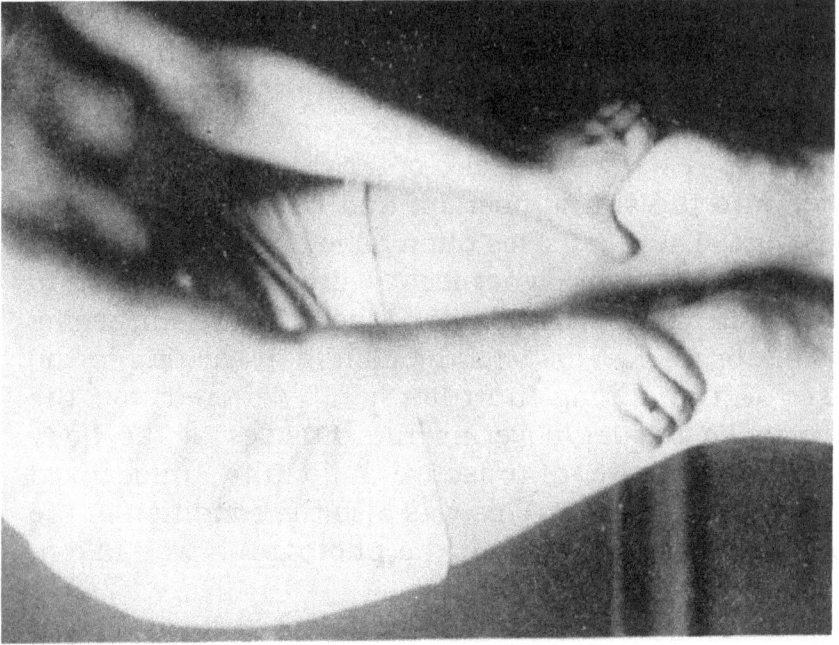

less important or less vital parts. We can live after amputation of a leg or a thigh, but head and heart cannot be dealt with in that way. But indeed a true view of the causes at work in the body shows how barbarous it is to recommend amputation of limbs and the removal of internal organs like the appendix or the ovaries when we have it in our power to advise patients to alter their conduct so that the causes of the ailments and disabilities of the several parts may cease acting, and the consequent conditions recover and disappear.

Figures 6a, 6b, 6c, 6d. (overleaf) The next two pairs of figures show pressure movements against the lower portion of the back over the false joints between the sacrum or expanded lower part of the spine and the iliac portion of the pelvis. It is called the sacro-iliac-synchondrosis on each side. The false joint allows of only a very slight amount of movement either in the forward and backward direction, or in rotation. But it is found to be stiff and tender in a great many persons, both male and female, as shown in the figures; and movement of it in the backward and forward direction with pressure is a good method by which the stiffness may be combated. Persons suffering in these false joints find themselves to ache when sitting down, but even more so when rising from a chair, and, not infrequently, more still in rising from bed in the morning. The exudation from the blood into the false joints appears to be deposited specially during rest or sleep. It is indeed partly in this way-that is, by elimination of waste matters from the blood-that sleep acts as a restorer of the body; and so, many persons are stiff when they come to move after having been asleep or after periods of rest.

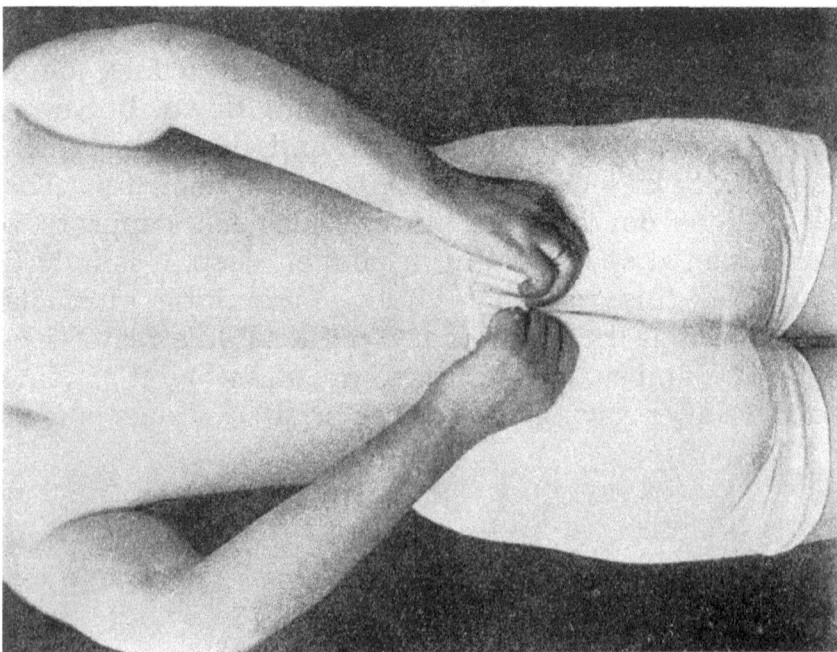

FIG. 6b

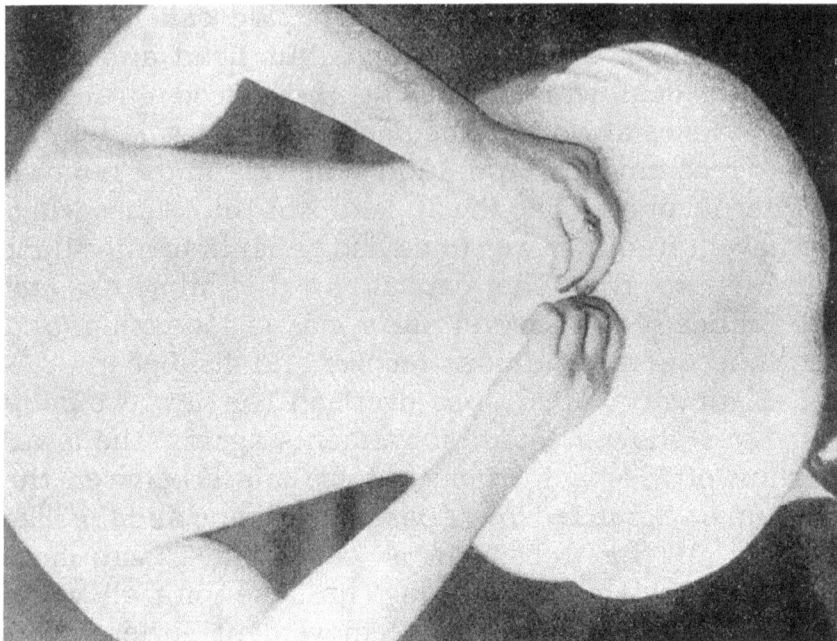

FIG. 6a

Self-movements under pressure of the False Joints of the Back (Sacrum) and the muscles of the Buttocks (glutei muscles).

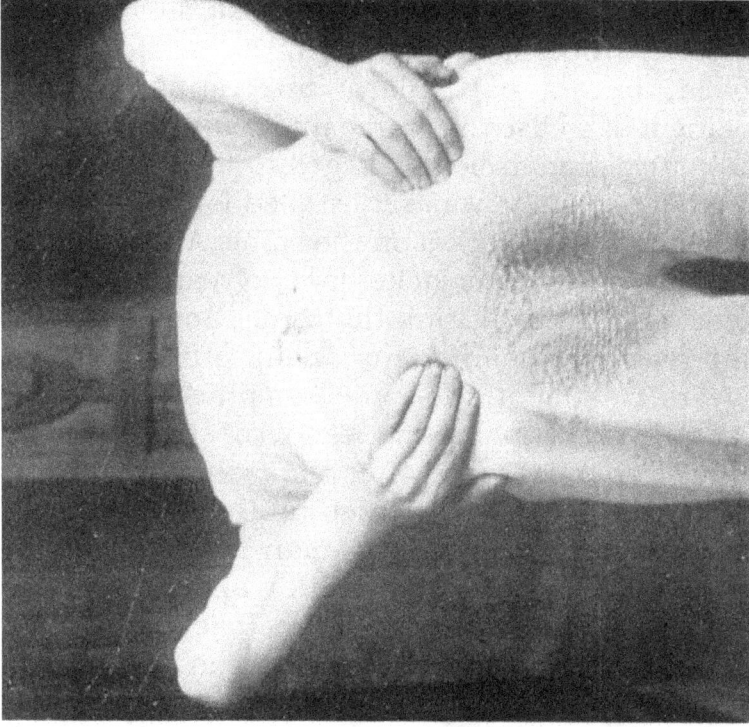

FIG. 6d

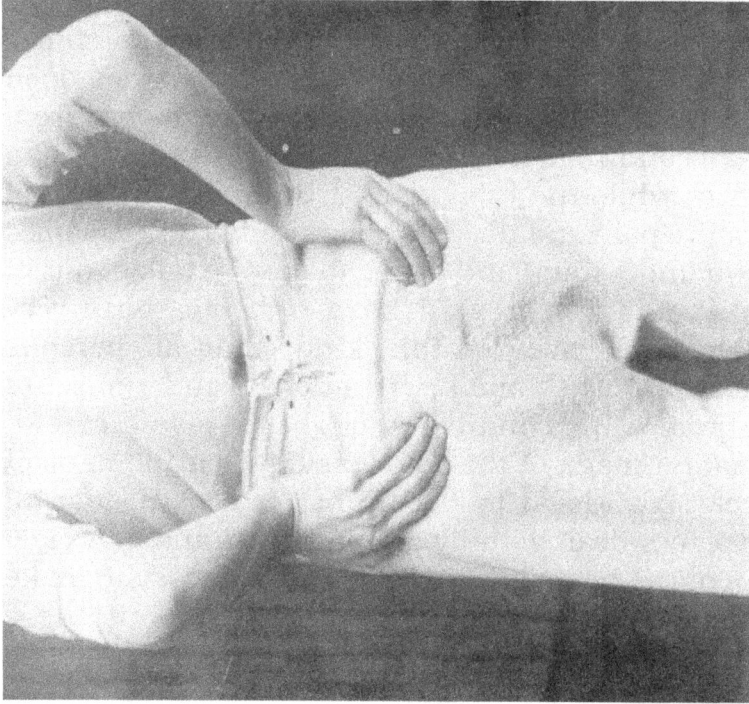

FIG. 6c

The same as 6 a and 6b.

115

Figure 7. This figure shows a position in which tenderness is occasionally found. It is apt to be overlooked, but is particularly interesting because overlooking it in a case that came under my observation led to a young woman being alleged to have disease of the spine. For this she was sent to bed for eight weeks with a plaster of Paris jacket on the spine. After that she had to wear a poroplastic jacket for two years. The pain was better and worse during that time. Sometimes for short intervals she was free from pain. Still at the end of two years' treatment, the spine was practically in the same condition of pain and tenderness as at the beginning. Under massage after the fashion shown in the photograph, partly by herself and partly with the help of her sister, the young woman in question has become well, and walks about briskly and with a light step. Not only is the extreme tip of the backbone (tip of the coccyx it is called) tender to pressure in such cases, but sometimes the ligaments attaching the bones to surrounding parts are so also. So indeed are the attachments of soft parts to soft parts, and sometimes in cases of this sort the act of having the bowels open sets up great pain from this cause. The misery from such a condition is more easily imagined than described; while the jubilation at being delivered from the obscure pain and the depression which accompanies failure to understand and disinclination to talk about it, is correspondingly great. I have come to think very strongly, from cases of this kind, that all persons suffering from "spinal irritation" and obscure "neurotic"or initic conditions, ought to have a careful examination made of the whole spine from the nape of the neck right down to the tip of the coccyx, and all tender places dealt with by manipulation and massage. Disease of the bone itself is comparatively easy to make out, and must be dealt with otherwise; but these ligamentous and periosteal and connective-tissue

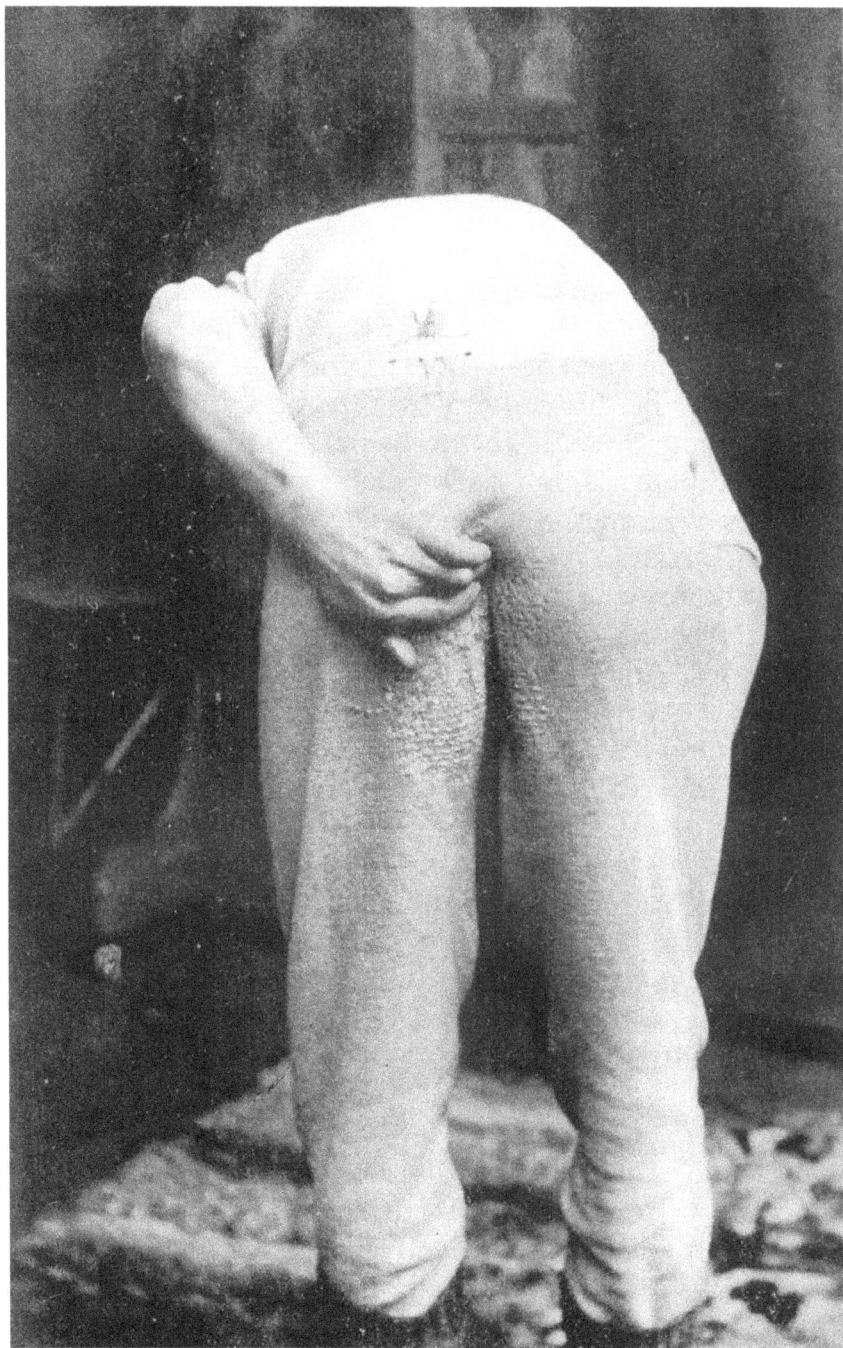

FIG. 7

Manipulation of the bottom of the Spine: tip of Coccyx.

117

conditions, though frequently obscure, often yield to treatment in the happiest way, and enable us when they are properly handled, to convert misery into happiness, and depression and despair into cheerfulness and hope.

The young woman who. was suffering from pain in this situation had had a very interesting although very painful history. She had been ill for eight years. When seven years of age she had had an abscess in the right side of the spine. This was thought to be perhaps due to disease of the vertebrae, but, as the case eventuated, it was seen to be due only to suppuration and necrosis of the connective tissue in the back, because, although a puckered depression was left at the place, no dead bone came away, and the wound healed quite soundly. The back, however, always remained rather tender, and no doubt the previous occurrence of the abscess made all parties who had to do with the case somewhat chary of dealing with it. It was no doubt safer to be too cautious than to be too rash. When, therefore, obscure and unexplained pain in the spine was complained of, it can be understood how disease of the spine was apprehended and even diagnosed. It is not to be wondered at, and yet it cost her some eight years of misery before the chief cause of her disability was reached, and being reached, was treated and cured.

Figure 8 shows manipulation of the inside muscles of the thigh, the adductors of the thigh as they are called, which draw the thigh to its opposite limb and are the means by which the one limb can be made even to cross over its fellow. These muscles, the adductors, longus magnus and brevis, with the gracilis muscle, are often very tender and that in both sexes, from congestion of the connective tissue covering the muscles, as also from congestion of the tendons of origin themselves from the pubic bone. Manipulation and movement is of value in removing the stiffness and tenderness and so restoring the feeling of lightness and

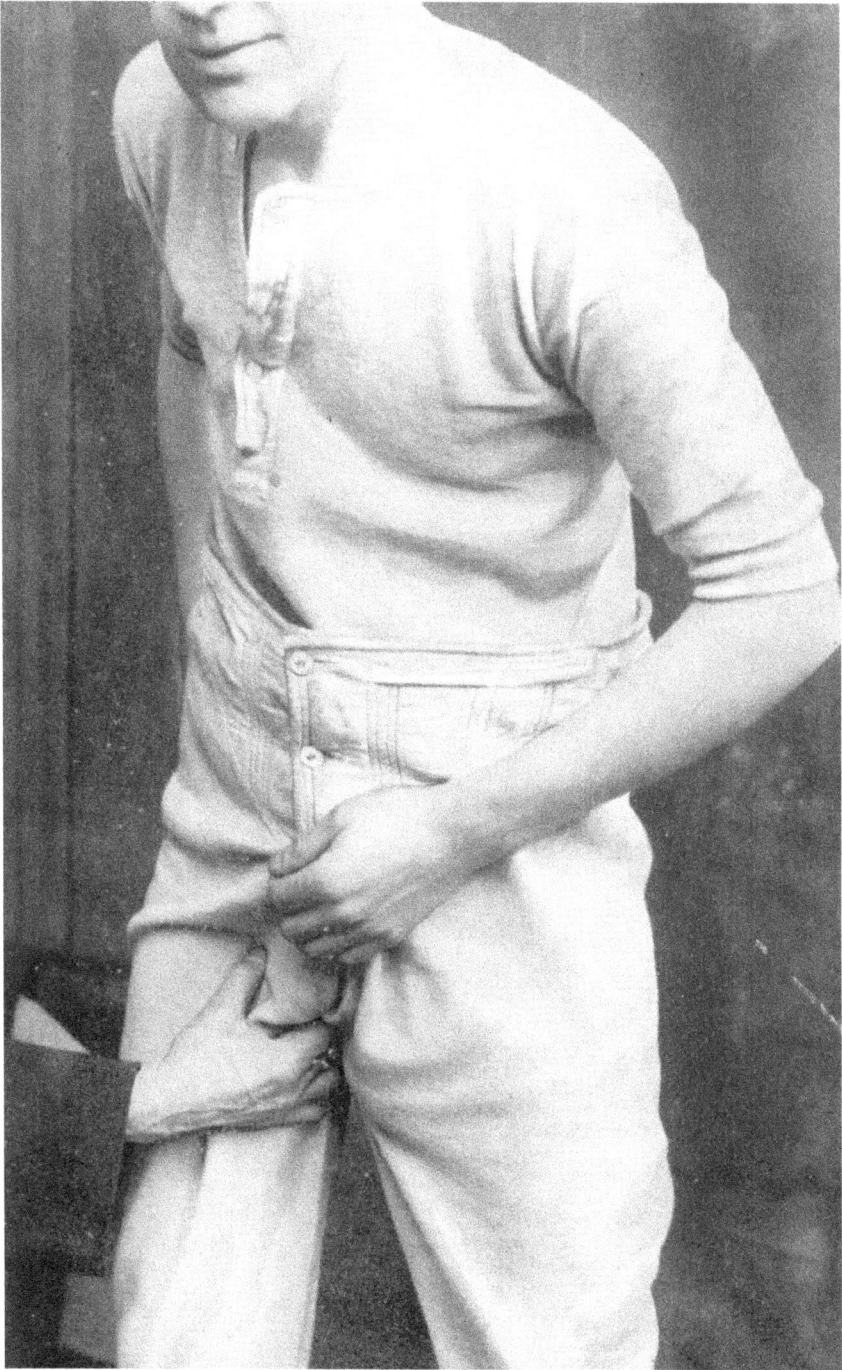

FIG. 8

Manipulation of the Muscles of the Inside of the Thigh: the Adductor
Muscles.

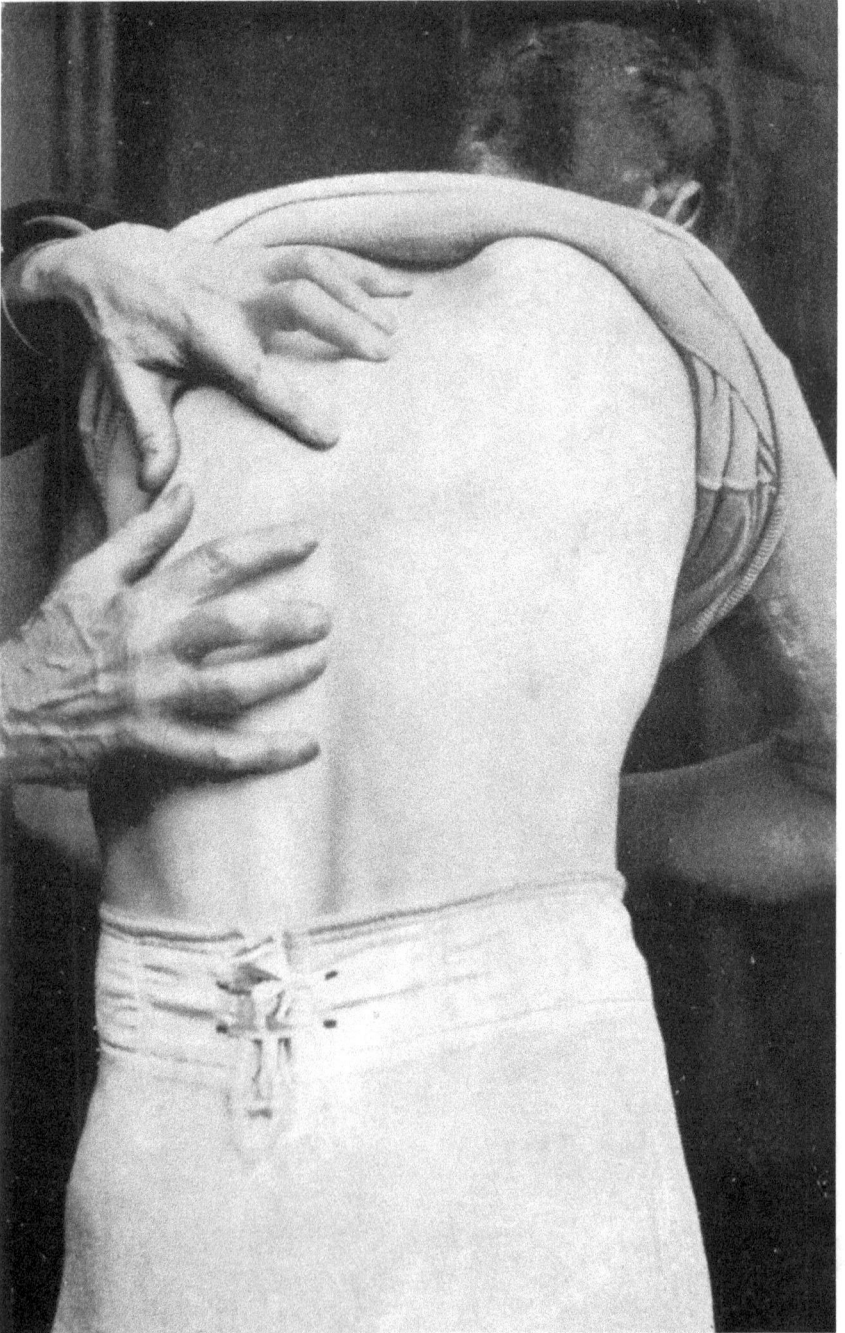

FIG. 9

Manipulation and movement of the Muscles of the Back: The Erector Spinae
Muscles.

freedom of movement, and removing the feeling of fatigue which so much oppresses patients who have often no idea how tender the parts are, or even that they are tender at all, until the tenderness is demonstrated to them by grasping the muscles. Of course both thighs ought to be moved and manipulated, as both are, as a rule, equally tender.

Figure 9. In this figure the hands of the masseur are shown pressing against the erector spinae muscles. These pass along the whole length of the back on both sides of the spinal column in a way that is at once simple and complex. From the nape of the neck and sides of the back of the head they pursue a simple general course to the firm bony pelvis at the bottom of the spine. But the intercurrent attachments to the various parts of the bony spine, as well as to the ribs, are numerous, and anatomists describe a sevenfold division of the erector spinae: muscle on each side. Harmony, ease and completeness of movement are obtained by this complicated arrangement of muscles and attachments. Incidentally, I may observe that it always appears to me difficult to explain how these and similar arrangements towards harmony and ease and comfort and efficiency are introduced. What is it that introduces them? Why should they be so well adapted to the attainment of their end, that end being apparently unconsciously aimed at?

As to the first of these questions, is not the proper answer that it is the force of life that is acting? If the force of life which accounts for the phenomena of plants and of animals were called bio-dynamic, then we should reply that bio-dynamic is the motive power by which phenomena harmonious to plant life and to animal life respectively are produced, just as, in order to account for chemic and electric phenomena, we assume a chemic force and an electric force, and a force of gravitation or hylo-dynamic to account for the phenomena of attraction. Bio-dynamic is a force more complex than any of these, although none of them is so simple as to be masterable without prolonged study; but bio-dynamic at once breaks up under examination into phyto-dynamic or the force that governs plant-life, and zoo-dynamic or that complex force which procreates, governs and accounts for the phenomena of animal life. And of course the particular phase of it under examination now is what we may call anthropino-zoo-dynamic or the force of human life. When I look at the phenomena from this point of view I confess to some difficulty in understanding the objection shown by scientific men to the assumption that a force of life or forces of life exist. Is it because they feel that a life-force or life forces can be only varieties of the universal energy by which all things do consist? But if so, what else is gravitation? Or what else is chemic force? Or electric force? Are not these also varieties of the universal energy? If the universal energy is itself alive, or if it is life itself in action in lower and higher forms, the difficulty seems to me to vanish. Of course this is not a scientific question but a philosophic one. But whether energy exists at all, or whether gravitation exists or chemic force or electric force, is, each of them, a question of philosophy also, and not of science, since each of them deals, not with facts but with the reasons which seem to account for them.

As to the second question, why should the arrangements introduced, say, in the complex attachments of the muscles of the back to the ribs and vertebrae, and the intricate arrangements and connections of the various fasciae and ligaments-how is it that all these arrangements should be so harmoniously adapted to use and comfort, and mobility and efficiency? Is it because this seemingly unconscious life-force is itself under guidance and direction? Is it the agent of a power, or does it emanate from a power that knows and adapts? The crude argument from design may perhaps have been superseded or the phase or form of it altered; but a more subtle and intricate form of it remains to be considered by the inquiring and candid mind. I deal with it no further now, for no doubt each reader and investigator comes to his own conclusion. If, however, all the forms of force are varieties of the one universal energy coming from the only source adequate to account for it, then no surprise need be felt if we find that they all work harmoniously. Their natural tendency is to the maintenance of order in what we call inanimate nature, and to peace, unity, harmony and happiness in what we call animate. As, however, animate and inanimate differ, as we have seen, not in kind, but only in degree, the natural effects of forces which are varieties of the one power by which all things do consist are order and happiness. Design need not be excluded, but even without design, order, happiness and peace are naturally secured.

To continue, however; the muscles of the back, intricately arranged and connected as we have seen, often ache obscurely over a greater or less extent of their course, and ought of course to be massaged all along their length and on both sides of the spine, although the illustration shows manipulation on only one side.

Figure 10. (overleaf) The next figure shows firm pressure being exerted by the fingers of the masseur (or masseuse) against the back of the shoulder-blade below the projecting spine, as it is termed, in what is known as the infra-spinatus fossa. This is very often—that is to say, in a great number of persons—a very tender place. As most persons are right-handed, the right infra-spinous fossa, as shown in the figure, is generally the more tender because a greater flow of blood in it occurs during its extra use. But of course the left shoulder-blade should be similarly moved and manipulated, because through anatomical arrangements and particularly through a bilateral nervous supply arising from parts of the nervous system close together, much sympathy exists between the two corresponding sides of the body. In this way good influences conveyed to the one are generally reflected to the other side. It is well, therefore, to manipulate both sides, even if one only seems to be affected; and this is a good general rule to follow in the treatment of any and every local disability.

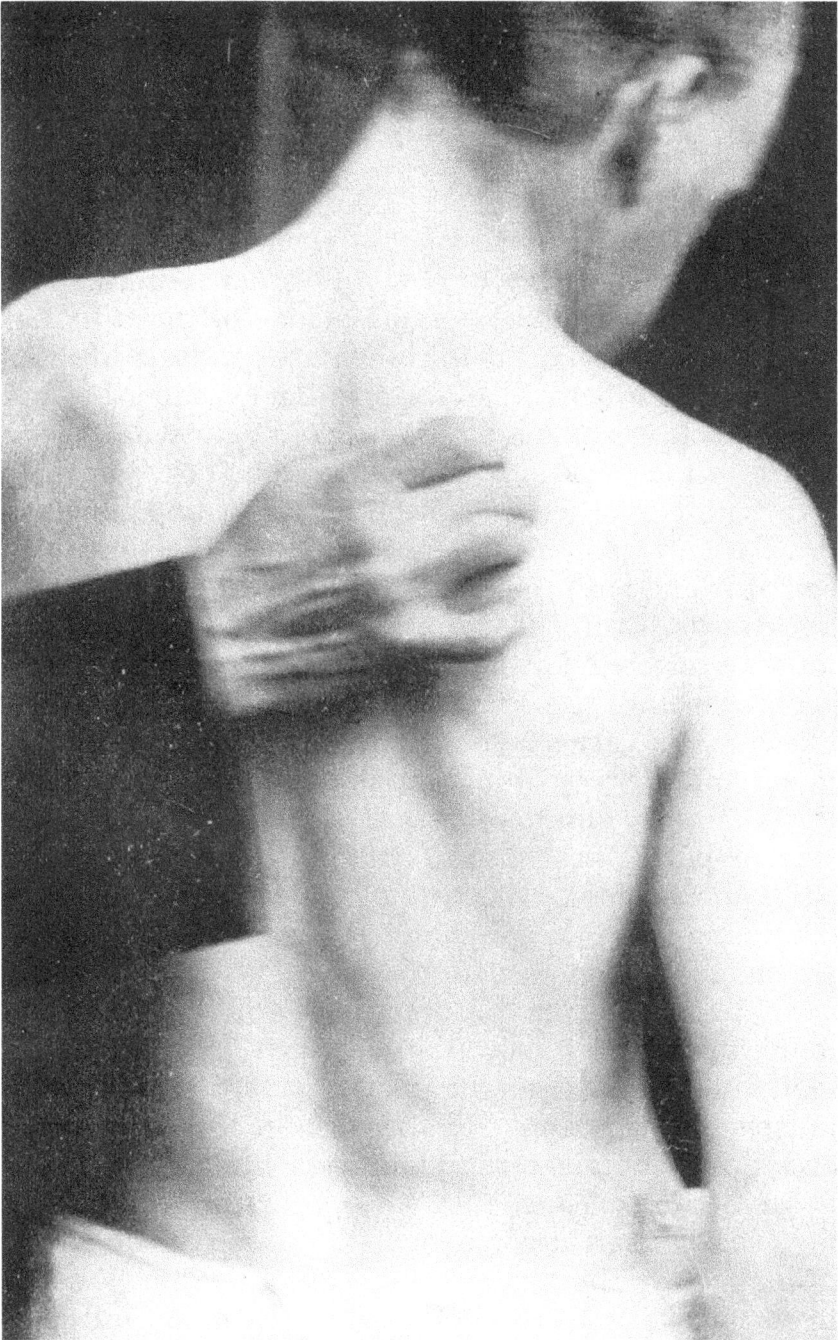

FIG. 10

Manipulation and pressure movement of the Infra-spinatus Muscle.

The infra-spinatus muscle arising from the infra-spinatus fossa, is not by any means the only one affected, although it is often the most tender. If, however, the arm be raised to the level of the shoulder, and there moved backwards and forwards, and if at the same time either the hand of the masseur or patient's own fingers are pressed against the back of the shoulder as if to oppose the movement, other muscles are generally found to be tender also. The teres minor muscle travels with the infra-spinatus muscle in order to reach the tuberosity of the arm-bone (humerus), and this muscle is also tender as a rule. And indeed so is the whole of the back of the shoulder. The teres major is attached to another part of the arm-bone and serves to draw it inwards towards the trunk, while the infra-spinatus and teres minor serve to rotate it outwards and backwards. Even these do not exhaust the list of the muscles affected, for the long head of the triceps muscle on the back of the arm is also tender in many cases likewise. The triceps here passes between the teres major and the teres minor on its way to reach the top of the shoulder. Anatomists must of course name the various parts affected, and without a dissection of the parts the names of the various muscles are apt to be confusing. To the layman, however, the general statement will soon be found to hold good that the whole shoulder is tender to pressure, and ought to be manipulated and moved in order to get rid of the tenderness. On examination, it is usually found that no muscle sheath escapes the congestion and tenderness; and it will generally be found that the back of the armpit is tender also; and this means that other named muscles, the serratus magnus and latissimus dorsi, are also affected. The names do not much matter. What is important is that the whole parts are tender, and have to be manipulated. The directions to masseurs and to non-medical people must therefore be that they should thoroughly manipulate and press upon the parts as patients are moving them, and especially wherever they may be found to be tender.

The infra-spinatus and teres minor muscles and others at the back of the shoulder and armpit are interesting in another way also, for they are generally affected with cramp and spasm, and by and by with wasting, in the affection known as writer's cramp. In the stage of cramp and spasm the writer's pen seems to jump and dart about as if automatically, and without the control of the owner. In the condition of wasting it is as if the pen would not write at all. In the early stages treatment is of the greatest importance and efficacy; but in aggravated conditions of the later stages the condition is incurable. This consideration affords another inducement to us to try to understand early what is going on in our bodies, with a view to its treatment and cure.

Figure 11. In this figure, pressure is shown as it is exerted by patient's own fingers on the trapezius or shoulder-raising muscle. If the person elevates the shoulder and continues the pressure, the tenderness is felt more. Continued and repeated movements of the shoulder up and down generally succeed in curing the affection—that is, the dull obscure pain and aching cease, and patient's movements become light and easy and comfortable and free from pain. As in the case of so many other movements, this one can be best effected either when the parts are uncovered, or when no more than a single layer of underclothing covers them. We cannot reach the parts easily when the clothes are on in the usual way during the day; and at least the coat or bodice ought to be removed when the movements are being performed. In doing this movement, pressure of the finger on the upper point of the shoulder-blade serves to show us how exceedingly tender it often is. Under repeated manipulation with pressure the tenderness can often be made to disappear.

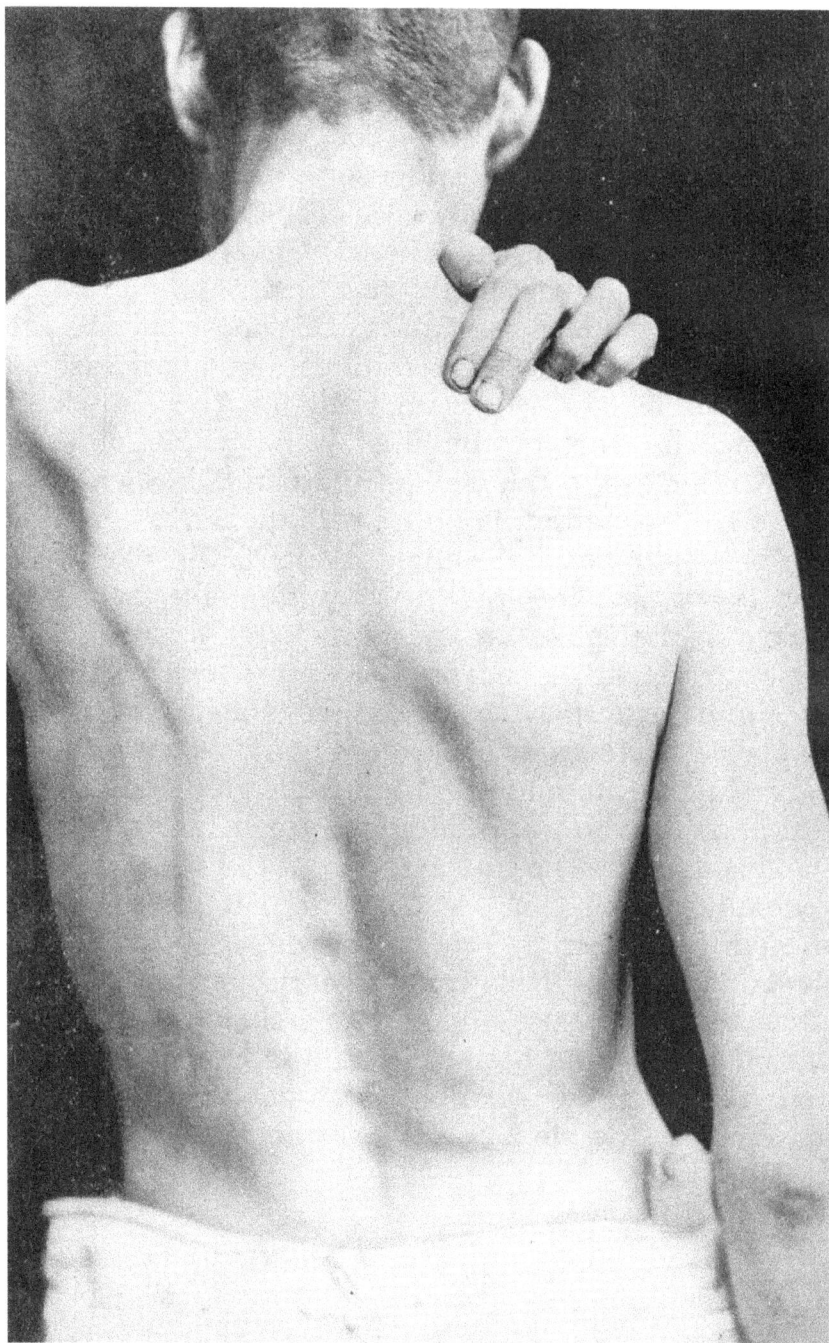

FIG. 11

Manipulation and pressure movement of the Trapezius or Shoulder-raising
Muscle.

Figure 12. This figure is intended to show massage of the muscles attached to the ilium (the anterior spine as it is called) or pelvic bone above, and to the fascia or strong connective tissue of the thigh below. These muscles are what are called tensores or stretchers of the vagina or sheath of the muscles of the thighs. They are often very tender, although perhaps not felt to be so till pressure is directed on to them. The buttock muscles, the glutei maximi and medii, whose sheaths are prolongations of the fascia in this situation are also as a rule found to be tender on pressure. These muscles pass to the part of the thigh-bone which projects outwards close to the neck of the bone, and which is called the trochanter. Pressure with the fingers into the soft parts just below the anterior superior spines of the iliac bones, and moving the body from side to side as shown in the figure, are measures often successful in removing the dull aching of these parts which translates itself into the feeling of being so tired. The fingers should be placed a little more backwards than is shown on the figure in order to massage the middle gluteal muscles. But patients who want to find out the aching places in the body, and who take the trouble to do so, will generally, in course of time, be able much to improve the wretched, depressed, fatigued feelings associated with the congestion of these connective tissues in whatever parts they may exist. Figure 12 is shown in *a* and *b* parts, to show that both sides should be manipulated, and also to show the obliquity and reversal of the movements suitable.

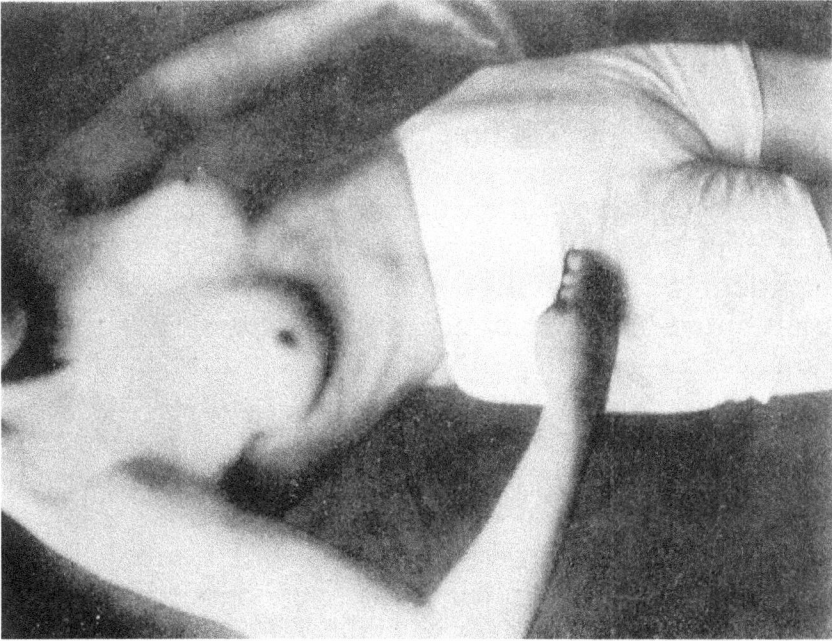

FIG. 12a

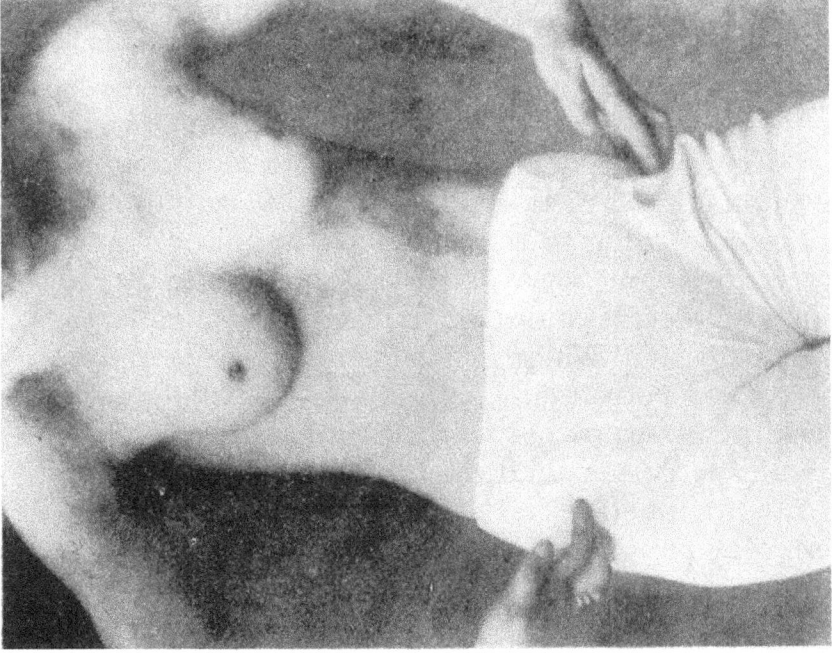

FIG 12b

Self-movements under pressure of the Muscles of the outside of the Hips; the Tensores Vagina Femoris; also of the Glutei Medii Muscles

Figure 13. This figure is also shown in an *a* and *b* form, and depicts a pair of movements which are very valuable in the treatment of ovarian neuralgia so called. The aching is referred by the patient to the side and front where the right hand is shown to be pressing in the photograph 13*a*. From what precise point the conditions leading to the sensation of pain or aching may spring is not always known by patients. Perhaps there is no precise point. That pain is felt is often all that can be truly said. *Where* it is felt is not a matter of direct sensation or perception; but judgment on that point is arrived at by a process of reasoning whose steps are generally forgotten; and, in fact, the judgment is not infrequently mistaken. That pain, therefore, should be referred by patients to certain places in the body is not sufficient proof that it really springs from those places.

What is termed ovarian pain often springs from the connective tissue about the back and not infrequently from that about the abdominal muscles; or at least is connected with congestion of these parts. Such pain or such symptoms in fact sometimes are found in men. Before resorting therefore to operation for the cure of such conditions, steady perseverance, or intermittent perseverance with movements should be persisted in for a considerable length of time, for a month or even three or more months. And in many cases the prosecution of general movements, and particularly of movements such as are depicted in this Figure 13, is followed by cure. The patient is shown with her left hand placed firmly on the left sacro-iliac-synchondrosis, while with her right hand she presses firmly into the oblique muscles of the abdomen. She then moves her body backwards and forwards with a slight lateral movement at the same time. This has the effect of moving the aching parts under pressure and of helping to remove the aching. Then the hands are reversed, the right hand being pressed against the right sacro-iliac-synchondrosis, and

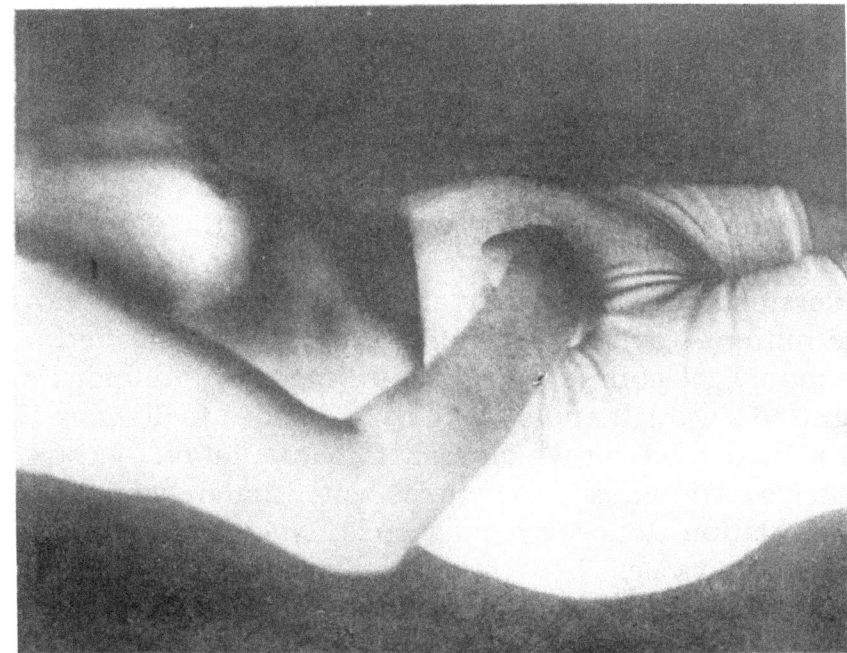

FIG 13b

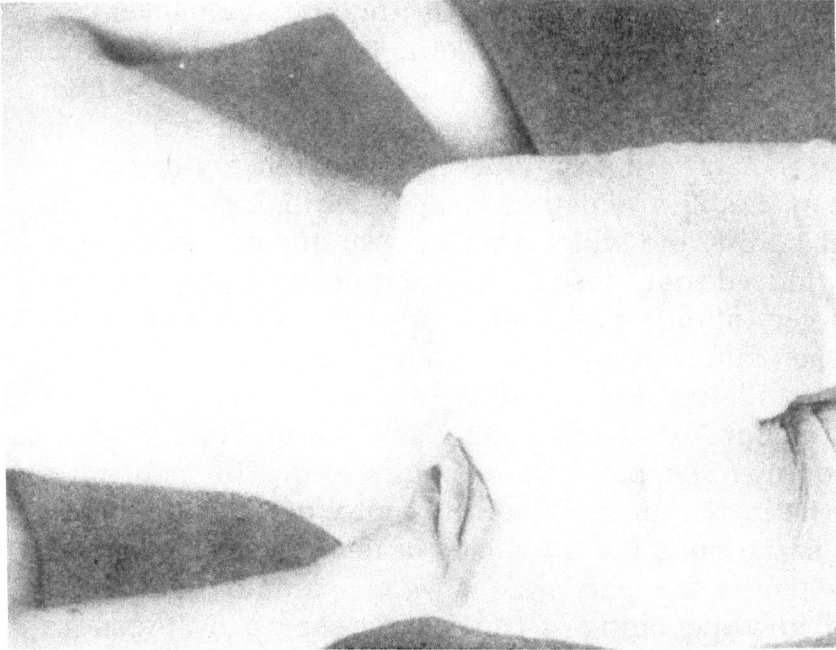

FIG 13a

Self-movements under pressure of the Side Muscles of the lower part of the Body, and of the False Joints of the Back (sacro-illiac-synchondrosis) simultaneously the left against the left oblique abdominal muscles, and similar movements carried out. Twenty-five or thirty of such movements on each side and repeated day after day, with perhaps half the number effected in the afternoon, afford a valuable means of relief and cure for the miserable and depressing pains which many women suffer from and which they find so difficult to localise. Not indeed that these pains are unknown in men—men are very often tender when pressed in the flanks—but women suffer from them far more than men.

In Figure 14, *a* and *b*, we see depicted another movement, the one I formerly said I often began with or recommended patients to begin with. The patient is shown to be manipulating the centre of the abdomen in the situation of the umbilicus or navel. It is astonishing how tender this part often is when examination is made and how sickening is the feeling set up by pressure there; and pressure of the hands into it with movement back and forward is very efficacious in relieving it. The manoeuvres have the effect of stimulating and of re-establishing the circulation of blood and of lymph in congested parts of the body and particularly in the passively congested parts of the digestive apparatus. As it is in the digestive processes and the apparatus concerned therewith that the foundations of these initio and rheumatic and quasi-neuralgic and myalgic conditions are laid, the rationale of the means recommended for their relief and cure can be easily understood; and when they are persevered with in the intermittent way recommended, cure is often effected. Obviously, of course, movements and manipulations might be so rough and so long continued as to do more harm than good, for which reason manipulation by the patient's own hands is sometimes better than having the manipulation done by a masseuse, since the patient herself knows best how much pressure she can apply without causing too much pain. Many masseuses are

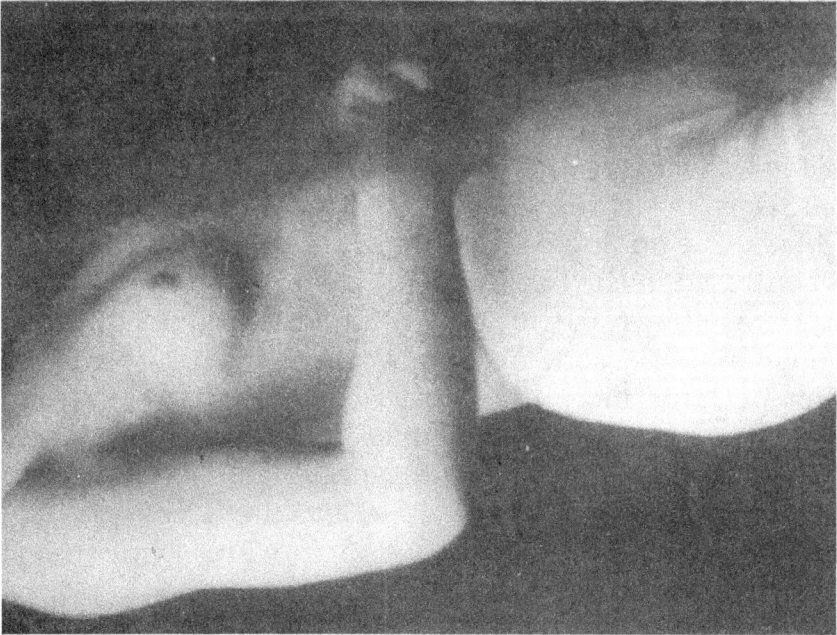

FIG 14a

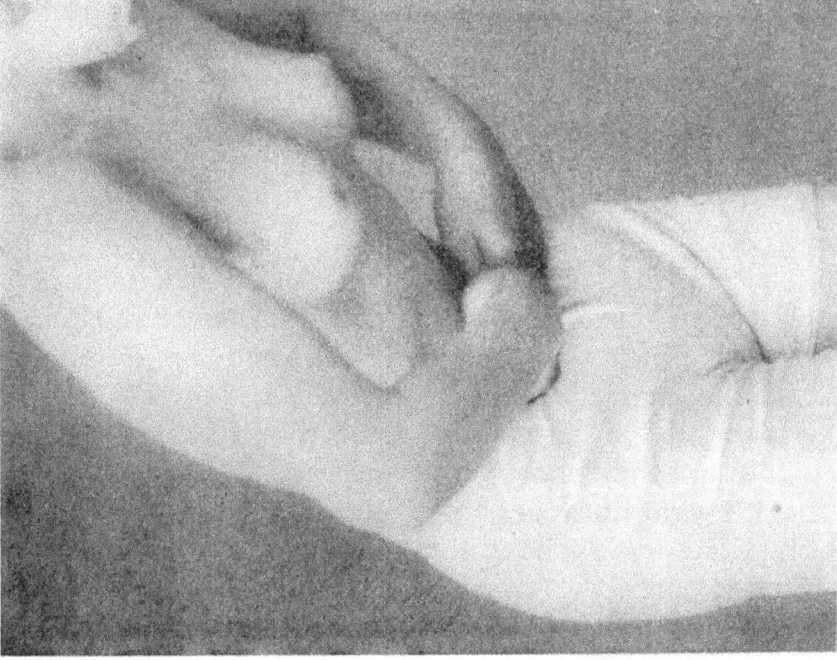

FIG 14b

Self-movements under pressure of the front straight Muscles of the Abdomen (Recti Abdominis Muscles)

now, however, skilled in applying these movements, and the presence of the masseuse is besides often a great comfort to the patient, who is frequently depressed by the obscurity of the pain and its indefinite and obscurely localised character. A combination, therefore, of personal movements with the help of the masseuse is often the best means of treatment.

In Figure 15, *a* and *b*, are shown movements adapted to remove or help in removing from the back of the neck congestions which lead to the aches and pains which afflict many persons, both male and female. It is true that many patients do not know that they have pain there, all that they know being that they do not feel well, or that they do not feel comfortable; and it is often left for the doctor to show them from what point the discomfort particularly springs, although no doubt it is more or less general. The whole connective tissue is tender and distressed, but in this particular place the distress is more than in most others. When patients suffer from megrims, or recurrent sick headaches, they are often tender if pressed in this region just where the head is attached to the neck and trunk. The aching can often be traced, or signs of it can be elicited, all down the back and lower limbs.

Very often patients who suffer from recurring sick headaches ache all the way down from the back of the neck, right down the lower limbs to the calves, ankles and feet. The aching being thus general, although more concentrated in the back of the neck, manipulation of it in the way shown in the figure affords a valuable means of relief. The person, man or woman (though women suffer perhaps more often than men in these ways, I have known many men who suffered also) presses firmly with the fingers into the tissues at the nape of the neck, what the Latins called the *nucha*, and the Greeks, ἰνίον. The head is bent backward and forward while the pressure is being exerted.

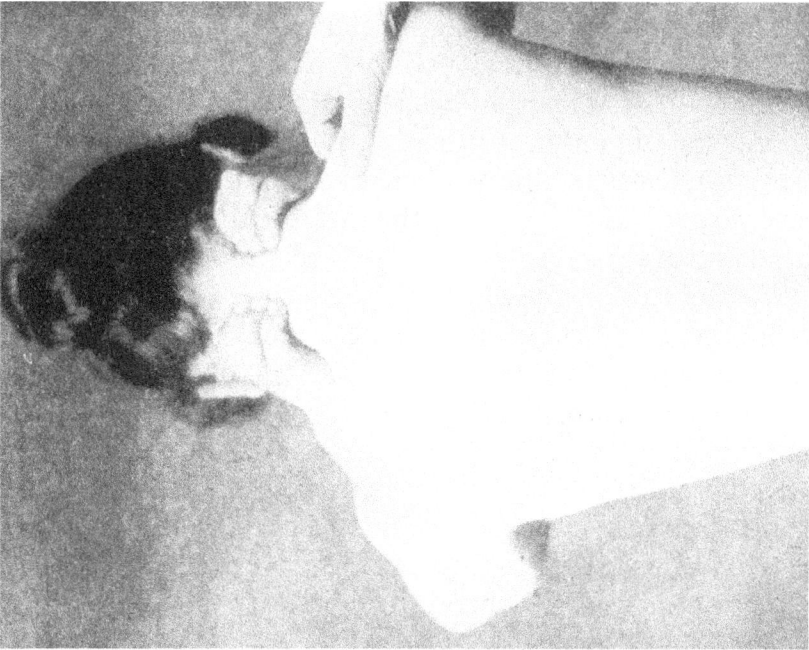

FIG 15b

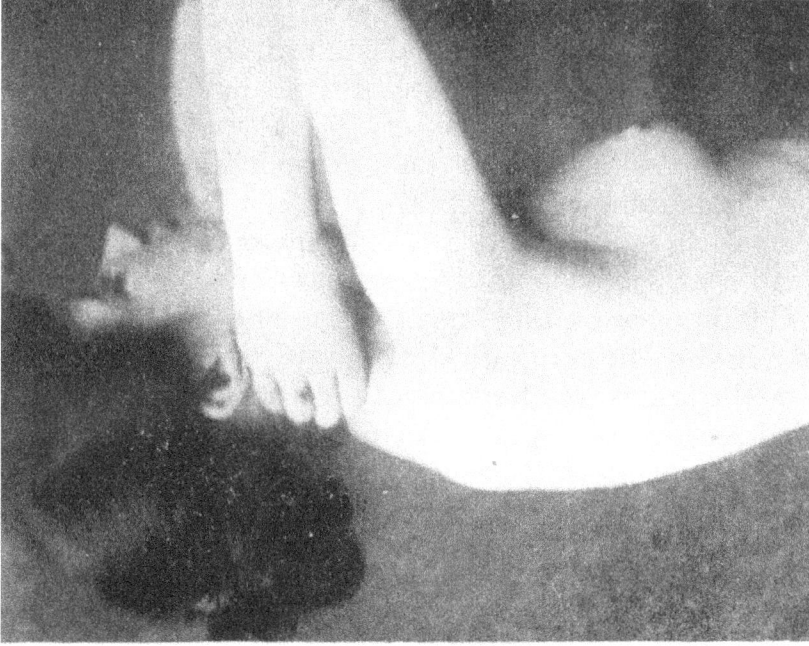

FIG 15a

Self-movements under pressure of the Muscles of the back of the Neck and Shoulder (Splenis Colli and Trapezius Muscles)

137

The hand of the masseuse is shown in 15a grasping the trapezius or shoulder-raising muscle, to show that it also generally participates in the tenderness. (See Figure 11, where the masseur is shown with his own fingers pressing against the corresponding place. This figure also shows how this place can be most easily reached in one's own body.) The side of the back of the head over the occipital bone is very often tender also; and tapping or patting this part of the head is efficacious in relieving the congestion.

The widespread extent of the congestion or of the tenderness from which we infer the presence of the congestion shows how ineffectual is the means too commonly used by patients of taking an aperient when one of these attacks comes on. The aperient can do little or no good. The two pills so often taken to relieve an attack of sick headache go so far no doubt towards the formation of the aggregate seventy-eight tons of aperient pills estimated to be taken in England annually; but we have not prevented our sick headaches by means of them, and neither have they enabled us to cure our constipation. Not infrequently sickness and vomiting set in, with the recurrence of these headaches, which is no doubt Nature's effectual manner of affording relief to the oppressed digestive organs. But even if there is no vomiting, there is almost always loss of appetite, so that, between the sickness and the compulsory fasting for a time. Nature sets about the relief of the affection in her own efficacious way. But we ought not to be so blind as to fail to see that it is the action of long-continued malnutrition, and really overloading of the digestive viscera that compels Nature, or the universal energy, one of whose forms is the force of life, to set up these periodic efforts to clear the system, and that it should be our business to see to it that the causes are no longer allowed to act-that is, we should recommend restriction of the diet, since it is through the mouth that the excess of nutritive material is introduced into the body; and we should also recommend the use of exercises to the pained parts. Repeated applications of counter-irritants like mustard plasters or mustard leaves to the back of the neck, every night for ten minutes for a week are also very helpful; but of course restriction of the diet is the main remedy, since it is the only one which goes to the cause of the malady.

Galen, who practised in Rome, dying in A.D. 200, and who wrote in Greek, said that recurring attacks of illness ought to be treated in the intervals and that we should not wait for the occurrence of the attacks. The Roman Emperor Antoninus Pius suffered from recurring attacks of megrim, which did not, it may be incidentally remarked, hinder him from reaching the age of seventy-five years. Galen probably had the emperor's case in his mind when he made his remark, although he was probably too young a man to be consulted about the emperor, who died in A.D. 161, when Galen was only thirty-one years of age. Be this as it may, however, many of those who quote Galen's views approvingly seem to do him little more than lip-service, for they do not put into practice the principles which they quote so admiringly. And so, many of the patients who suffer from recurring ailments to-day, recurring headaches, recurring colds, recurring attacks of influenza or of asthma, etc., are no more philosophically or wisely treated than were patients 1750 or more years ago, for in nearly all cases we wait for the occurrence of the attacks, rather than attempt to obviate them by proper treatment. We say that prevention is better than cure. But we act as if we really believed that cure is better than prevention. It is true unfortunately that patients themselves are not particularly anxious to have the causes of their illnesses pointed out to them. In cases where they suffer from recurring headaches they prefer, many of them, the prescription of two aperient pills and a bottle of medicine. And in cases of recurring asthmatic attacks they do not like to be told that, as the lungs arise in development from the digestive tract, and as their immediate purpose is to rid the body of CO_2, which is a product of the digestion, the true and best means of treating asthma and recurring colds and bronchitis is by restriction of the diet. But although these things are so, and although it is often a rather thankless task to try-for prevention rather than for cure, it is still a question what the duty of the medical profession is in the circumstances. Each member of it will, I suppose, act in accordance with his judgment and his conscience and no more is to be said.

There are great rewards in effecting cures and relief from suffering and in adding to the length of life on one plan; and there are other rewards on other plans. Nature, however, is very long-suffering with us and behaves very mercifully to us. Generation after generation the force of life continues to act and to reproduce the race. We are not swept away, although both we and all our ancestors break, and have continued to break, the laws of life and health for an indefinite number of generations. If disease were hereditary and cumulative, how could we have survived? True, one set of diseases does seem to be hereditary, and, in three or four generations, strains that are the subject of sex-crimes do seem to be swept away from off the face of the earth, do what we can for them. It seems as if the perpetration of sex-crimes was the unpardonable sin from the physiological point of view. But even here the strain being swept away, the race goes on without it and is not infected by it. The main charge against us of the human family is that we do not pay sufficient attention to the tragedies that overtake us and that we go on, are too apt to go on, breaking the laws of life and of health as our predecessors did. In the other cases, and as a general rule, what seems to happen is that our lives are short and full of suffering, that our days are few and evil; as indeed, how could they be anything else in the circumstances?

Marcus Aurelius, who succeeded Antoninus Pius, died at fifty-nine years of age, not because of the hardships of the campaigns which he carried on against the Quadi and the Marco-manni, as historians tell us; but because, Galen not with-standing, he did not understand nutrition. Waking, as he often did, at three o'clock in the morning, and wisely betaking himself to study then rather than to using various sleeping draughts, he unwisely ordered a breakfast at that early hour, and struggled with the labour of digesting it while his brain was labouring as the instrument of reading and writing. But this was not all; for as his father by adoption expected him to breakfast with him at eight or nine A.M., he took another meal then, and then another about midday, the *prandium*, as it was called, finishing with the court dinner, or the *coena*, at about eight P.M. Could he have known it, it was this late meal which was the immediate cause of his waking at the very early hour he did. If he had eaten nothing after the one PM. meal (*prandium*) he would have had a much better chance of life, and in the course of a very few days he would have ceased to wake at a too early hour, but would have slept right through the night. As it was, he died at the deplorably early age of fifty nine, the hardships of the campaign no doubt contributing to it, but the main or predisposing causes being the choking of the body with so much food "to keep his strength up," no doubt) as lowered its resistance so much that it was unable to contend with the hardships of the field.

The warning which might have been taken from this history has had very little effect on other rulers, or, for that matter, on other men and women since. The late King Edward the Seventh, of gracious memory, appears to have had a double broncho-pneumonia, for which he was treated, and we are assured with great benefit, by the hypodermic injection of serum elegantly made from his own sputum. He died at sixty nine years of age, on a Friday, the immediate exciting cause of which sad event seems to have been a dinner-party to which he insisted on motoring on the Monday of that week, although he felt shivery at Sandringham on the Sunday. At any rate, when his physician saw him on the Monday night, his pulse and temperature were quickened and elevated, and he died on the Friday. At about the same time I was advising a poor man who had suffered for many years from double broncho-pneumonia. He was sixty three years of age, not quite so old as the King. I advised him to take one meal a day, about midday, and he did so. He had no serum injections to withdraw his attention from the real causes of his illness; but he is living yet in comparative or fair health; and I have little doubt would have been in better health still, if he had begun treatment ten years sooner than he did.

It is tempting to pursue this subject, because the food habits, not only of royalty, and of the nobility and well-to-do portion of the community, but of the poorer classes also are so deplorably destructive of health. There are hardly any of us so poor as to be unable to get too much food. On the other hand, we might have thought that the subtle intellect that evolved the "Thoughts," that sage and beautiful culmination and acme of the stoic philosophy and ethics, might have shown more insight into health matters, but apparently it did not. But the eminence of men in one direction of knowledge is no necessary guarantee to their eminence in another or in others. We have seen before that men may be eminent in science and yet be very indifferent in philosophy; and now we see that a man may be great in philosophy and even in spirituality and yet be weak in the ability to read his own physiological nature; for it is difficult to believe that Marcus Aurelius did not suffer from discomfort or fatigue from his wrong food habits. Thus he writes:

"This morning I got up at 3 o'clock and after a good breakfast studied till 8."Again : "I slept late this morning on account of my cold .... Then I gargled my throat." How modern it all is, and how we learn from these letters of the great emperor to his beloved tutor Fronto the similarity of the ailments, and the similarity of the causes of the ailments, from which humanity has suffered in ancient and modern times. And Pliny the Elder, who perished in the volcanic eruption at Herculaneum in A.D. 79, was too "wheezy" and stout to escape, like so many modern men at fifty-six years of age who do not understand nutrition, or, if they do, do not allow their understanding to sway their conduct. Fronto himself, we read, suffered from gout !!

And yet there is no evidence that he ever imagined that the true source of his suffering was that he took too much food, any more than the same reflection occurs now to the vast majority of his successors on the earth. But if, generation after generation, men have had the same lesson put before them and if we have refused to learn, whose fault is that? Nature's? Or Fate's? Or our own?

As for Commodus, the son of Marcus Aurelius, and brought up with all the care which the noble mind and ample means of his father could supply-let us not talk of him, but look and pass on. If young men *will* destroy the inheritance laid up for them by their fathers or predecessors, no power in nature will say them nay. That is not the method of Nature's government. The consequences ensue: that is all. And if the younger generation of an old nation do the same; if they say that the child alone matters, the consequences will come too, and that swiftly. For one thing, when they who are the children now become the fathers and mothers of the next generation, they will still be apt to think that it is

143

themselves who matter most. And this may wake up their children's minds to see that selfishness is hateful in whomsoever it appears, and that self-restraint and consideration for other people are higher qualities than self-indulgence. The next generation may therefore tend to be more cautious and wise and self-governing than its predecessor, and so progress and improvement may for the time being be seen. It is, however, rather disheartening to observe how, generation after generation, nations seem to forget or to fail to benefit by the lessons of their own history. We seem so slow to learn and so apt to pervert the teaching which the revolution and revelation of nature seem unceasingly to be setting before us. If we have it insidiously suggested to us (without its being said, of course) that it is easier to vote for wages than to work for them, that the idle are to help themselves perforce to the reward of the industrious, and that amusement and not work is the chief end of life-well-is not the nation that votes such advisers into power, and especially the youth of that nation, liable to be corrupted ? Even Galen himself only reached seventy years of age, although some say that he lived to one hundred and forty. Suidas, I believe, is the authority for what is probably the more accurate statement.

Figures 16a and 16b and 17a and 17b show manipulations by the person herself of the front of the armpit and of the back of the same. It is desirable to have the clothes off, or to have only a thin layer of clothing on, in order that the parts may be properly reached and manipulated. The parts are frequently very tender on pressure, the back wall perhaps more so than the front one, though both are so. In number 16a and 16b the great and small pectoral and chest muscles are moved and manipulated at the same time. In number 17a and 17b the latissimus dorsi muscle, the infra-spinatus and the teres minor and major muscles are

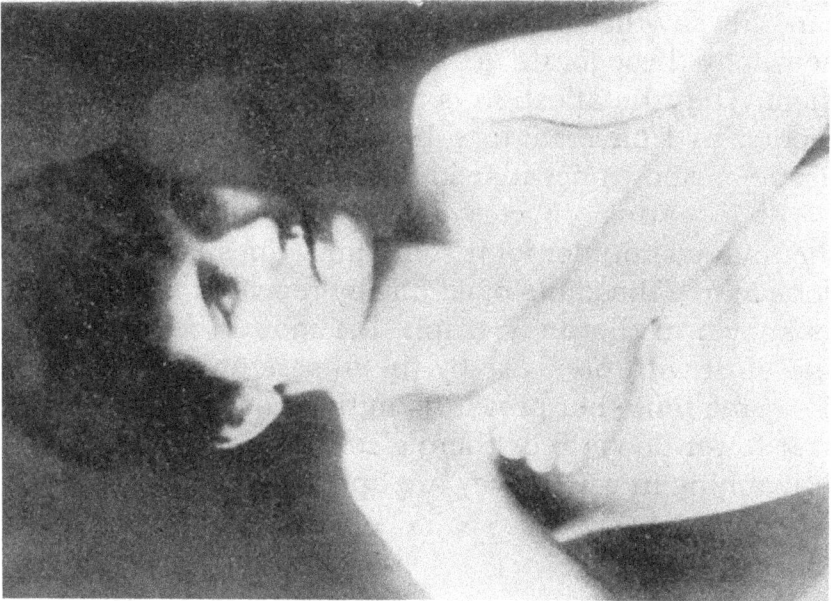

FIG 16a

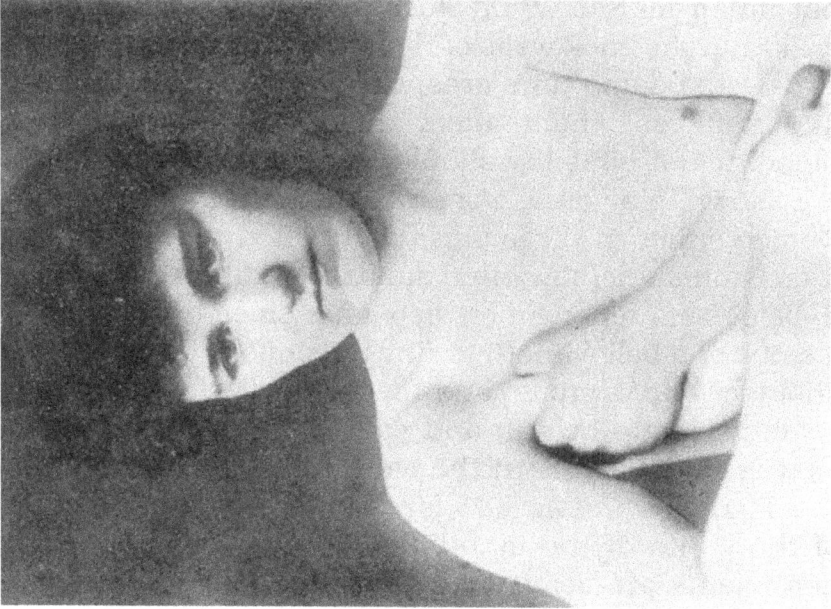

FIG 16b

Self-movements under pressure of the Muscles of the front of the Armpits (Pectoralis Major and Minor Muscles)

145

manipulated and moved. The names of the muscles do not much matter. What does matter is that the front walls and the back walls of the armpits should be moved and at the same time grasped so that the tenderness and stiffness which affect them and interfere with mobility and pliability should be removed. These parts are shown in a young woman. I think on the whole that women suffer in these parts more often than men; but it is astonishing how often similar conditions are found to be present among men also. Many men cannot throw a stone or a ball without feeling uncomfortable about the shoulder and armpits, and these muscles are found on examination to be stiff and painful, or at least tender, as well as the others at the back of the shoulder.

Figures 18a and 18b (overleaf) show manipulation of the joints of the mandibles at the same time that movements are being effected in the parts. These jaw-joints are often very tender. Many people (women more especially but men also) ache when they eat or ache when they talk, the aching proceeding from the congestion which is so often present in these joints. I can only say that it is a continual surprise to one to find how achy these joints are when examination is made of them. That the affection is rheumatic (but rheumatism seems, as I have said, to be congestion of connective tissue) is shown because in a minority of cases the jaws clank in eating, in very much the same way that a rheumatic shoulder joint sometimes does. Much can be done to free the joints of aching by repeated movements, as shown in the photograph, the mouth being opened and shut with pressure by the fingers on the joints, at the same time that pressure on the masseter muscles a little lower down frees them also from the stiffness and dull aching in which they are apt to participate.

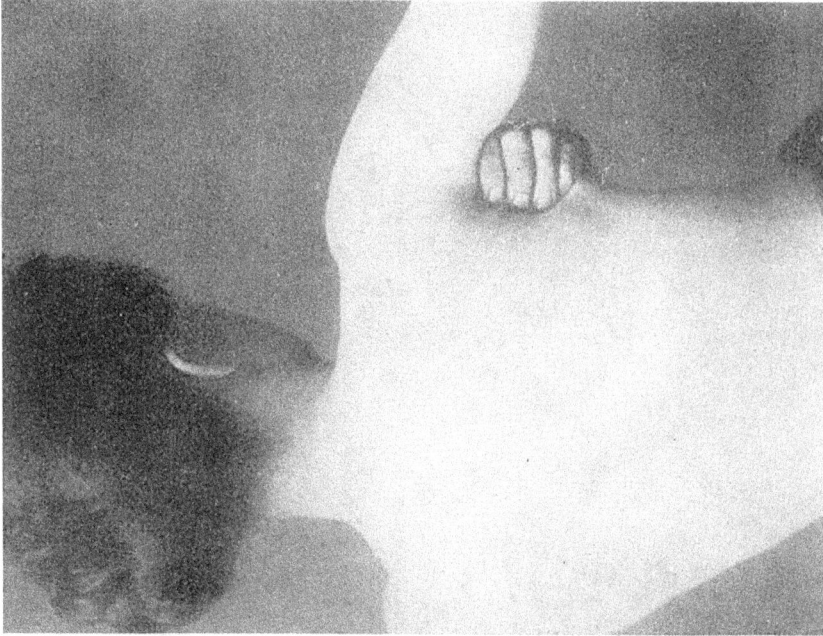

FIG 17a

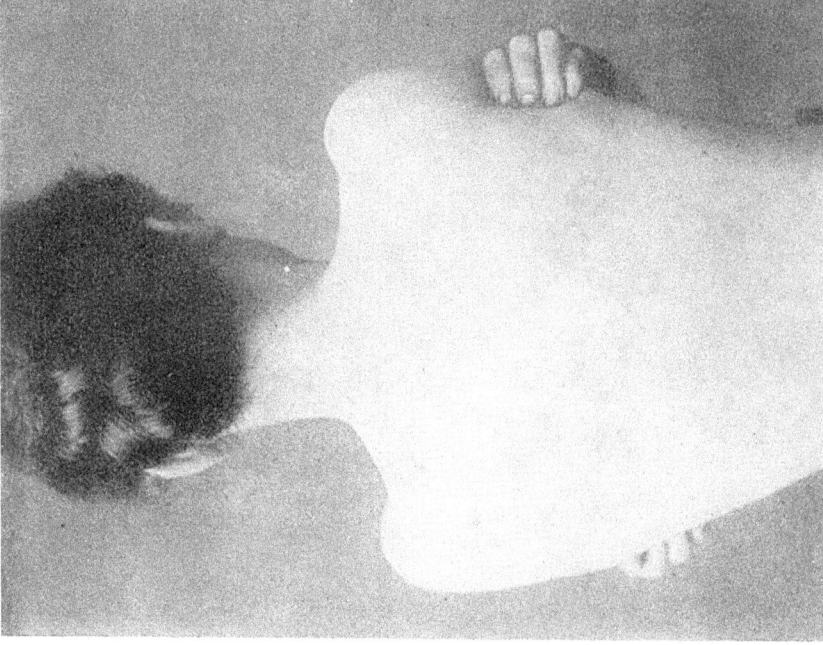

FIG 17b

Self-movements under pressure of the Muscles of the back of the Armpit and Shoulder (the Latissimus Dorsi and Infraspinatus Muscles)

147

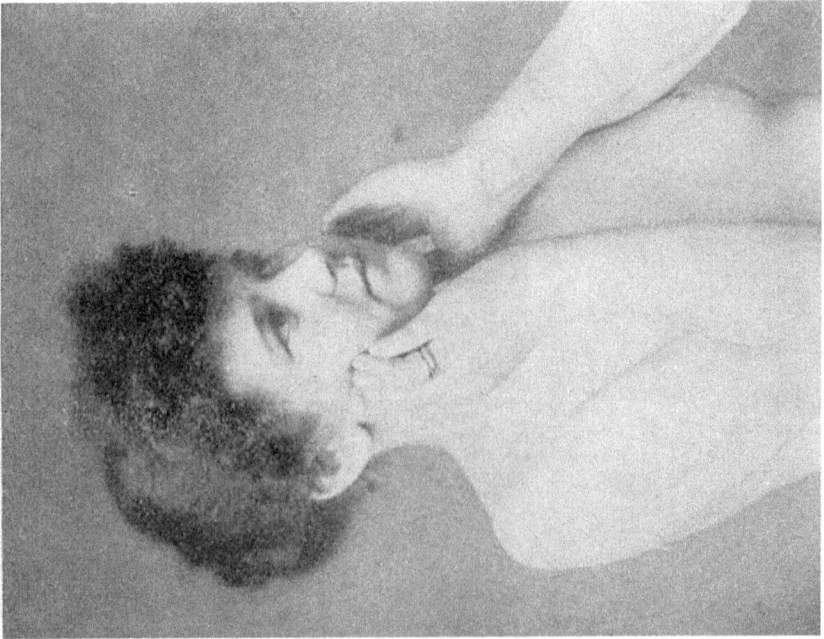

FIG 18a

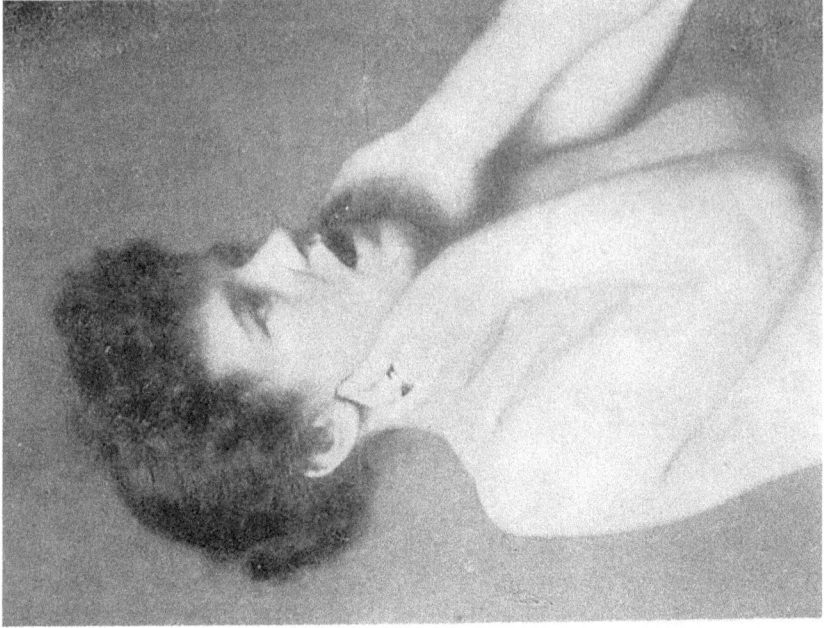

FIG 18b

Self-movements under pressure of the Muscles of the Joints of the lower Jaw, and of the Masseter Muscles

Figure 19 (overleaf) shows a pressure movement of the sterno-mastoid muscle which is often accompanied by aching and tenderness. These muscles on each side pull the head downwards and forwards and to its own side, and on both sides manifest the tenderness on pressure which we have now seen to be so common and whose general or even universal character and presence is so important in showing what is going on in so many cases in the human body. Twenty-five or thirty movements effected twice a day, or even once a day, do much to relieve and dissipate the congestion and to restore lightness and freedom of movement. The patient finds out just how much pressure can be borne by the grasp of the fingers and thumb, while the movements of pulling the head downwards and forwards by each muscle to its own side are being effected; and the repetition of such pressure movements removes the aching and congestion. Of course, the muscle on each side of the neck ought to be treated, although one only is depicted.

Figure 20 (overleaf) shows pressure movement directed to the sternum or breast bone. As the sterno-mastoid muscles last dealt with are attached to the sternum, we naturally follow the bone down and in doing so find out, often to our surprise, how tender it is. The breast-bone is, like other bones, covered with connective tissue or periosteum. It is also divisible into three parts with a false joint between the upper and middle part or body of the bone and another between the body and sword-shaped lower end. On examination the tenderness is found to be progressive from above down, that the bone is less tender at the top, and more so, often a good deal more so, over the centre of its body. The lower part of the body of the bone and the sword-shaped or ensiform lowest part are often very tender indeed. As the tendons of the pectoral muscles which form the front wall of the armpit stretch on each side on

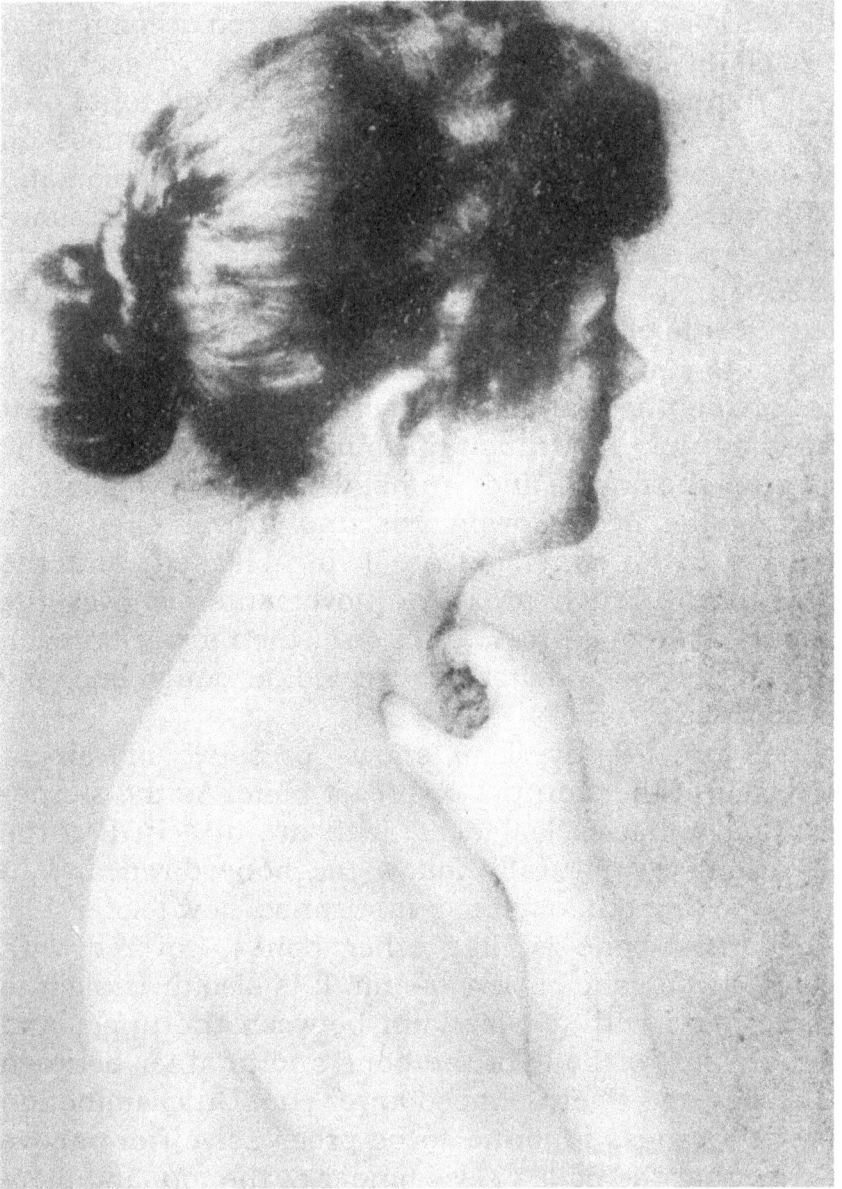

FIG 19
Self massage of the Sterno mastoid Muscle

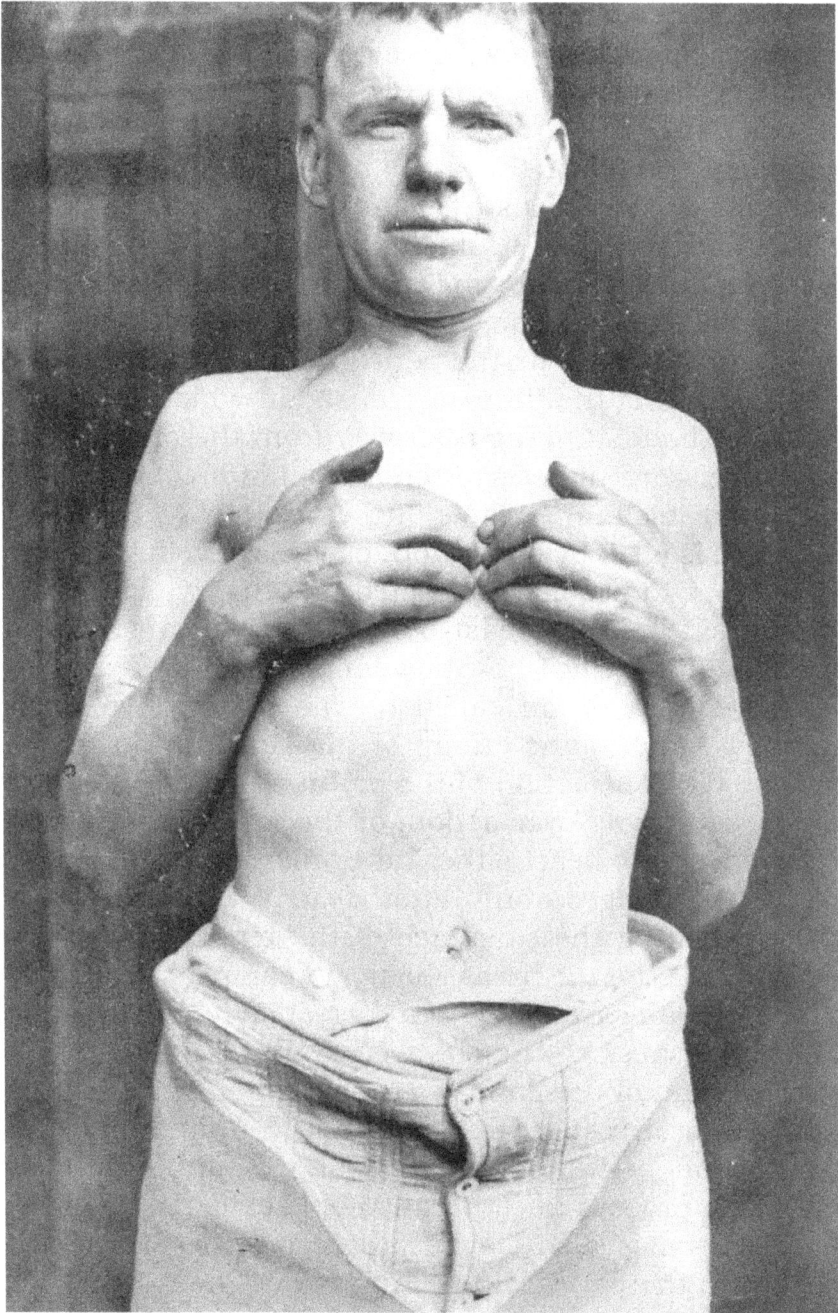

FIG 20

Pressure movements to the Sternum or Breast-bone: to prevent attacks of Angina Pectoris

to the breast-bone, the significance of its tenderness becomes more apparent, since it is seen to be connected with the tenderness which we have formerly seen to characterise the pectoral muscle sheaths. But more significant still does this appear when we find that from the under or interior surface of the back of the breast-bone there pass two ligamentous bands.[1] These spring from the upper part or manubrium of the breast-bone, and from its lowest or ensiform part respectively; and their purpose is to fix the pericardium in its place. The pericardium is the fibro-serous sac in which the heart lies, and bands finding their way from the breast-bone to the pericardium exert therefore an indirect action on the heart itself. The whole of the space just under the sternum is filled by mesh work of connective tissue, and this is apt to become congested like that which covers the outside of the breast-bone where we can reach it with the finger and show how tender it is.

In the condition called *angina pectoris*, which is usually a rheumatic cramp of the heart, a too strong spasmodic contraction of the organ may put an end to life by setting up over-action, or the inhibition formerly referred to; the heart either never dilating with diastole at all, or doing so only after death. If, therefore, by demonstrating the existence of the tenderness of the outer surface of the breast-bone, we can reason our way to the probable existence of a corresponding congestion and tenderness of the connective tissue on the inner surface, and of the bands which go to the pericardium, how important it is that we should understand the connection between the two. For no doubt the slow insidious process affecting the connective tissue of the breast-bone is also slowly progressive in that which passes to the pericardium. Further, as the nutrition of these parts leads to their slow blocking, no doubt the nutrition of the heart itself is coincidently affected by the process which is proceeding over the whole body at once and simultaneously. Irritant waste products carried by the blood will be likely to set up over- stimulation and over-contraction of muscles anywhere, and therefore of the heart muscles also. In these ways a fatal attack of *angina pectoris* or rheumatic spasm of the heart may occur. On the other hand, repeated manipulation of the periosteum of the sternum, by relieving the congestion of its reachable parts, will have a correspondingly beneficial effect on the deeper unseen structures, and by freeing and lightening them will prevent serious and possibly fatal developments. For these reasons, much more importance ought to be attached to tenderness over the sternum than it usually receives, since its occurrence is co-incident with important changes occurring simultaneously in deeper and vital structures, and particularly because good management of the parts within reach has a very beneficial effect upon the more important ones out of reach. I feel sure that proper treatment has prevented the occurrence of many fatal cases of *angina pectoris* in persons whom I have seen. It is a very important matter, because these cases are mostly fatal, and because there seems reason to think that the fatal termination can often be prevented, or at least postponed for a long time, often for years.

Figure 21(overleaf) Similar reflections occur from examination of the conditions shown in Figure 21, where the fingers of the man are pointing and pressing on the articulations between the breast-bone and the fifth and sixth left ribs. These are just over the position of the heart, although separated by the pericardium intervening. For some reason, I suppose on account of the presence of the heart on this side, the articulations between the sternum and the left ribs are generally much more tender than the corresponding ones on the right side.

Manipulation of the tender parts has the most helpful influence on the general nutrition and in

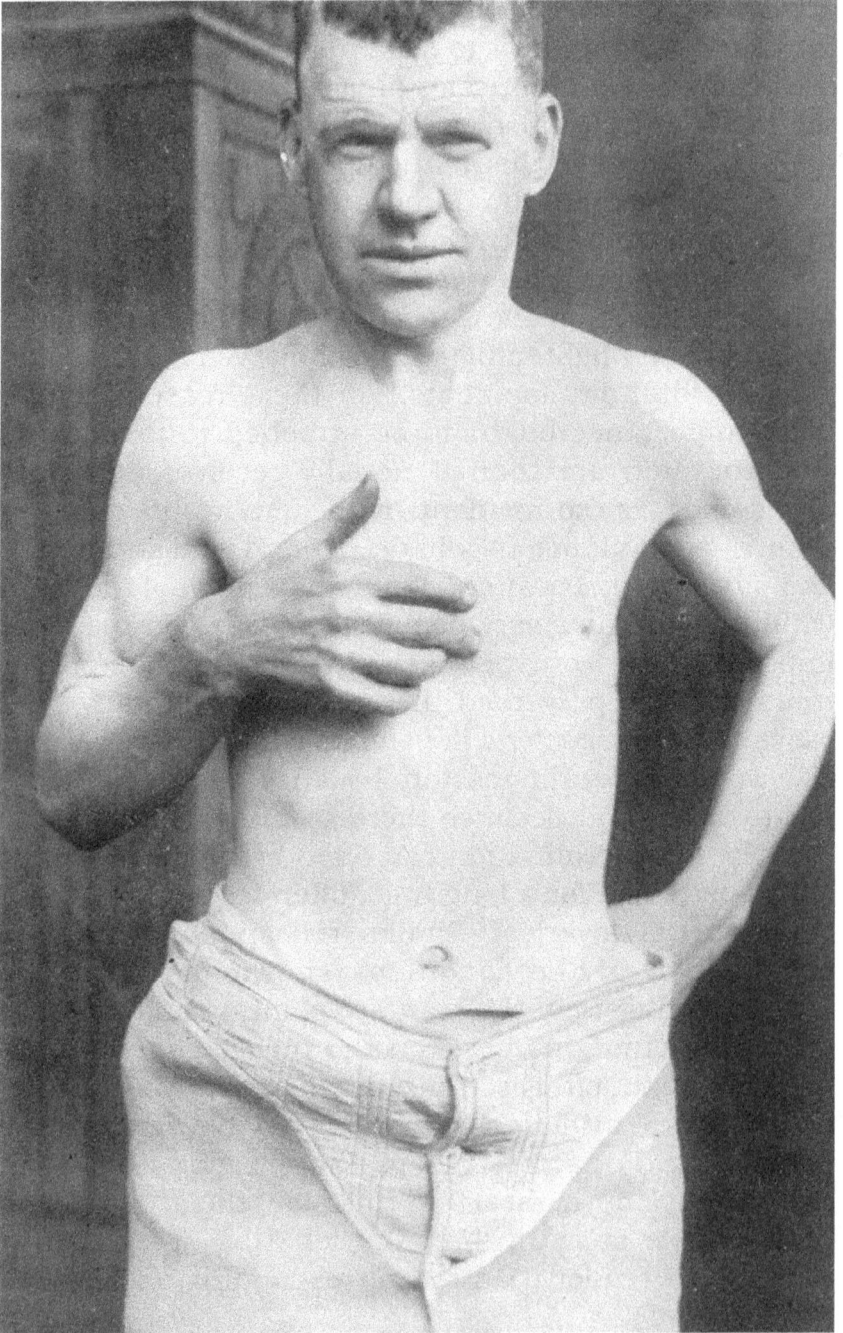

FIG 21
Self manipulation of the Articulation between the Breast-bone and the 5th
and 6th left Ribs, in order to prevent attacks of Angina Pectoris

154

removing tenderness from the whole region. I have no doubt at all that in quite a large number of cases I have been able, by directing the attention of patients to what was going on in their bodies, to prevent attacks of fatal angina by enabling them to cure themselves. This may perhaps be difficult to prove; only the occurrence of death in fact would prove it; and the price is far too high to pay for winning in an academic argument. Even if death does occur, and if it occurs as predicted, it is always open to the critic to say that the explanation given of the event was not the true one, so that there is no satisfaction derivable from this sort of argumentation. But I have in my mind two cases of this sort, one in a man of sixty-eight and one in a woman of sixty-five, in both of which I feel certain that death would have occurred from *angina pectoris* if attention had not been directed to the tender places, the exceedingly tender places, present, and if appropriate treatment had not been adopted. Both of these persons are living still. If we do not open our eyes to what is going on, it is certain that we shall not see.

The cases referred to are not the only ones I have seen where death has in my opinion been prevented, and that for years. Most of the patients of whom I think this has been true have been Elderly-that is, over fifty-five, while some have been over sixty-five; and I can think of some who died before I realised what was going on in their bodies. But when we look at the whole condition of the connective tissue and see how it is being affected all over the body, year after year after year, it seems very easy to understand how the slow and insidious process begins and goes on even from early years, and how it is apt to culminate in disaster after fifty or fifty five. The statement, therefore, so often made that "you cannot prove it," is not very disturbing. Probable evidence is a very important form of evidence, and is all we have or can have to go on in many of the most important situations in practical life. It seems to me particularly strong in this kind of case, so strong as to have entirely convinced me. Suppose the sceptics acted as if it were sound evidence, and adopted the treatment. It could do no harm and might do good. Suppose they gave it a trial. The unqualified people will certainly do so and make fortunes out of it, if the qualified profession do not. The clinical nexus and sequence formerly referred to when it was said that *angina pectoris* often followed on general and special initis have, I think, been emphasised by a further examination of the facts. The reader should make up his own mind, for his health and life are at stake and depend on the conclusion he comes to and the steps he takes to carry his conclusion into practice.

Figures 22 to 27 deal with manipulative movements of the upper extremity. In Figure 22*a* and 22*b* the patient is shown manipulating the shoulder, and particularly the deltoid muscle. The right muscle is shown and is most commonly affected, mainly, I think, because most persons are right-handed; but of course both shoulders should be moved and pressed and manipulated. The deltoid muscle (so called because its shape it resembles the Greek letter "delta," a character with a triangular shape) raises the arm upwards and outwards from the body until it reaches a right angle; and it is also the means by which the arm is moved both forwards and backwards. The muscle can be felt contracting if the fingers of the opposite hand are pressed against it when these movements are being effected. It is often very tender, especially at its back and front borders. It is the muscle, or one of the most important muscles, used in throwing a stone or cricket ball. It is also used in writing, along with many other muscles, the triceps on the back of the arm, the biceps and brachialis anticus on the front, and the muscles of the fore arm, etc. It is therefore apt to be affected

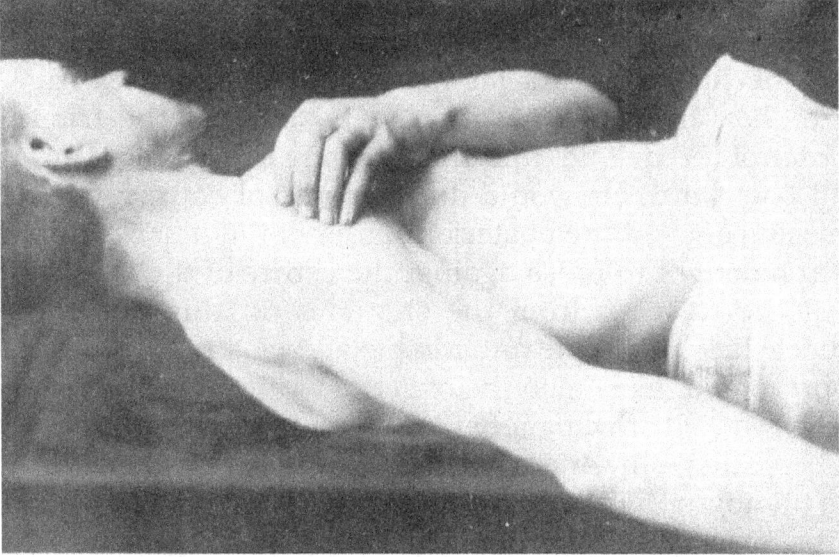

FIG 22b

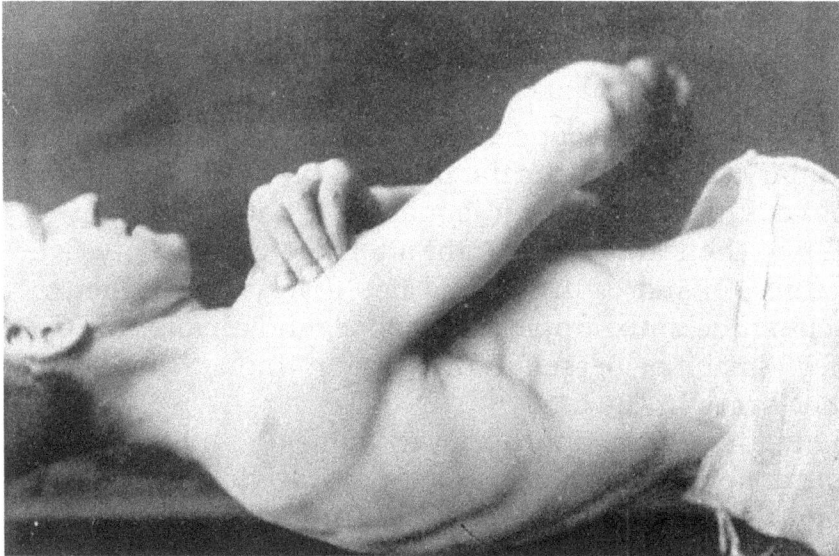

FIG 22a

Manipulation of the Shoulder and Deltoid Muscles

157

somewhat in writers' cramp, although not so much as the other muscles of the arm. But attention to it and proper exercising of it is very valuable as helping to prevent (among other things) the onset of writers' cramp,

The figure speaks for itself. The man is pressing with the fingers of the other hand against the front border of the deltoid, and then moving the arm forward and backward. He would do the same of course when pressing against the posterior border of the muscle; and then he ought to press against the centre of the muscle while he raises it from the shoulder. In this way the muscle is kept supple and pliable and elastic; stiffening is prevented, as is also the onset of writers' cramp; and the power of throwing a ball or stone is retained.

Another movement for the shoulder not shown in the photograph is to hold in the hand a handled ewer or water vessel and to rotate it by letting it swing as far as the hand and arm can be made to turn round, and then letting it turn or rotate in the opposite direction. Much of the rotation is obtained by the action of the shoulder muscles, the deltoid, triceps, biceps, teretes, infraspinatus, latissimus dorsi and pectorales, etc.; but some of it is obtained by rotation of the radius which carries the hand on the joint where it articulates with the humerus or arm-bone at the elbow. A housemaid's ordinary pail will do for the purpose very well. By taking hold of it by the handle it is made to rotate from right to left and then from left to right alternately for twenty-five or thirty or more turns. This has a very good effect in keeping the limb supple and mobile, and anyone can do it for himself or herself in dressing in the morning or at other times in the day.

Figure 23a and 23b shows extension and flexion or contraction of the triceps muscle at the back of the arm, while it is held and pressed by the performer's other hand. Flexion or bending of the elbow accompanies extension of the triceps, while extension of the elbow as

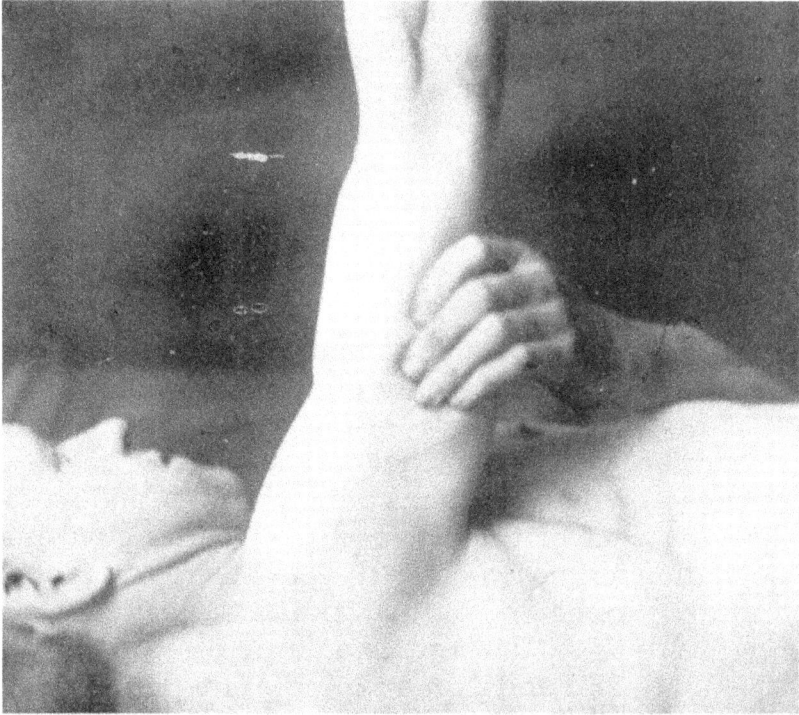

FIG 23b

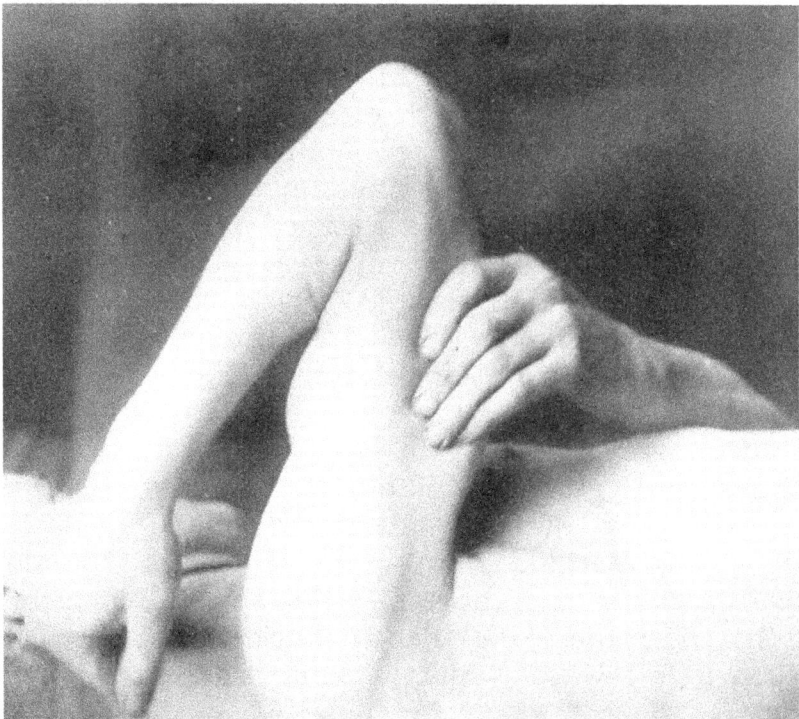

FIG 23a

Manipulation of the Triceps Muscle on the back of the Arm

shown in 23b accompanies flexion of the triceps. It is a very useful manoeuvre to keep the parts mobile, and should be repeated twenty-five or thirty or more times once or twice a day.

Figure 24a and 24b shows movement with manipulation of the elbow joint. The thumb is pressed against the inner side of the elbow while the joint is flexed or bent as shown in 24a or extended as shown in 24b. This inner side of the elbow joint is tender, and sometimes even very tender, in many persons who have no suspicion of what is going on in their bodies. The muscles whose action bends the fingers take their origin here; and fatigue and—disinclination for movement is experienced by many persons who are quite unable to localise the seat of their disability. This fatigue and disinclination for movement can be greatly relieved, and even entirely removed, by manipulation of the elbow twenty-five or thirty times twice a day.

In Figure 25a and 25b, rotation of the fore arm is shown, while the muscles attached to the outer. condyle of the humerus or arm-bone are being grasped and pressed. It is a very valuable movement, and brings into notice the extraordinary and often quite unsuspected tenderness of the parts. The neck of the radius itself shows this feature very strikingly, patients feeling not only discomfort when it is grasped but often even positive pain. They will often flinch very much under this manoeuvre while they bear many others with comparative indifference. The fore arm is shown in rotation in two positions, extension and flexion. In 25a and 25b (overleaf) the elbow joint is in extension. In 25a the thumb and lingers of the opposite hand grasp the muscles springing from the outer condyle of the arm bone, while the hand and thumb are rotated inwards. In 25b the fore arm is shown in the act of being rotated outwards, the back of the hand being shown. When the limb has been rotated further the back of the hand will be turned downwards while the palm will be turned up.

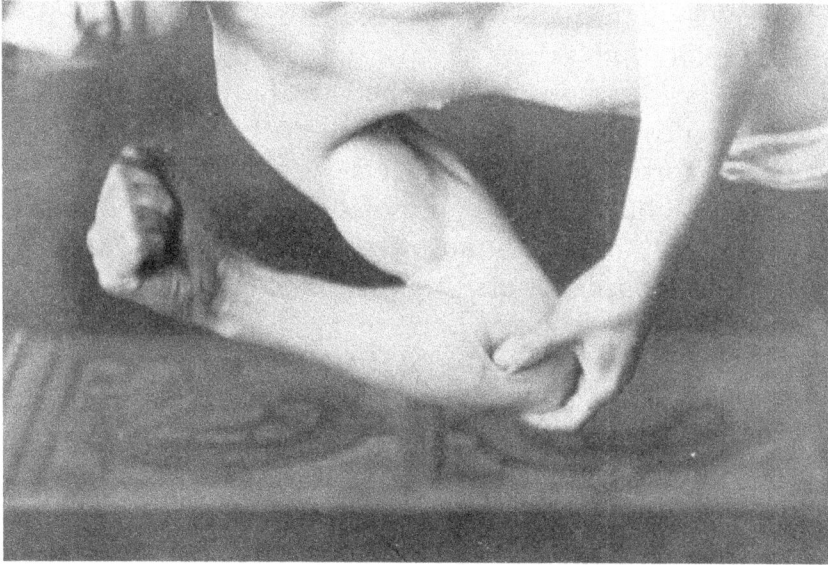

FIG 24a

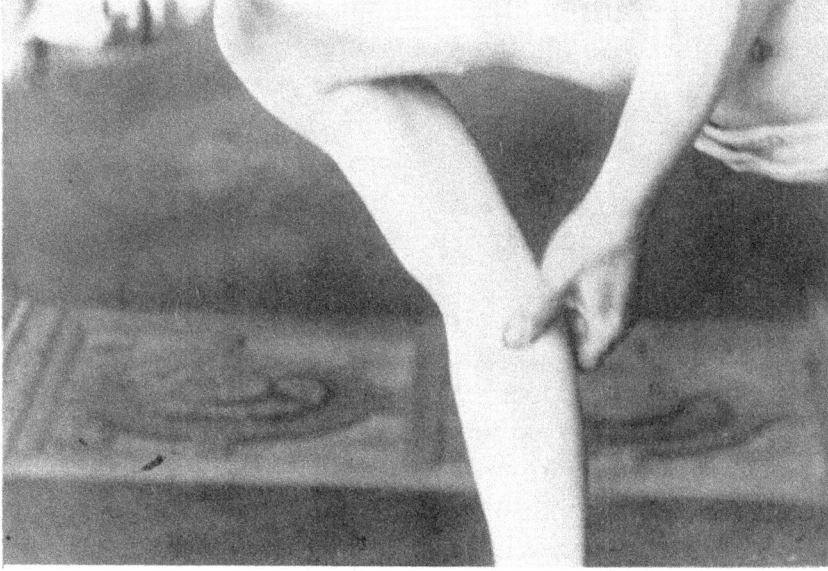

FIG 24b

Manipulation of the Elbow-joint particularly of the inner side

In 26a and 26b the same movements and manipulation are shown while the elbow joint is in flexion. These are valuable movements by means of which mobility and pliability can often be restored to the elbow joints.

In Figures 27a and 27b flexion and extension of the wrist joints are shown. This joint is often tender on pressure, although not so much or so often as some other parts; but movements under pressure are valuable in preventing the joint from becoming stiffened, and immobile, and in preserving its elasticity and usefulness. There are no fewer than eight bones described as going to form the carpus or wrist, and when we remember that, besides these, the radius and ulna, the two bones of the fore arm, enter into its composition also, and not only so, but that the five metacarpal bones carrying the five digits of the hand likewise articulate with the wrist joint, we may have some idea of the complication and also of the importance of the joint. No fewer than fifteen bones thus enter into its structure, and as they articulate with one another by gristle or cartilage, and as the joints are lined by synovial membrane, and attached by numerous ligaments, while many tendons are either attached to the joint or glide over it, lined by their synovial or peri-tendinous sheaths, one may form some imperfect idea of the very complicated character and important functions of this joint. It is truly marvellous how seldom so complicated a piece of mechanism gets out of order, and how long it lasts. In this last respect, however, perhaps the reader will ask himself whether the length of its duration as a useful piece of machinery is anything like as great as it ought to be, or as perhaps it will be when its owners understand nutrition, and, understanding it, allow their conduct to be swayed by their knowledge.

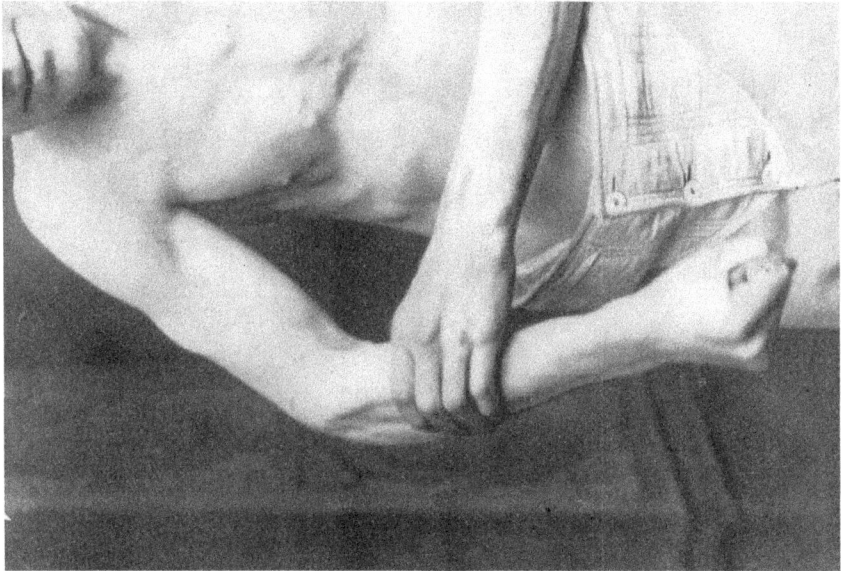

FIG 25b
The Elbow is in Extension

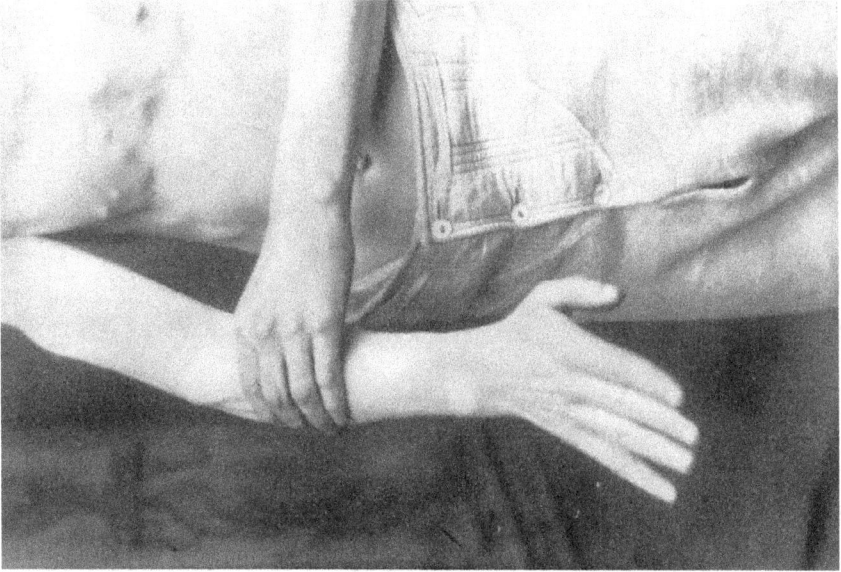

FIG 25a

Manipulation of the Extensor Muscles of the Forearm.

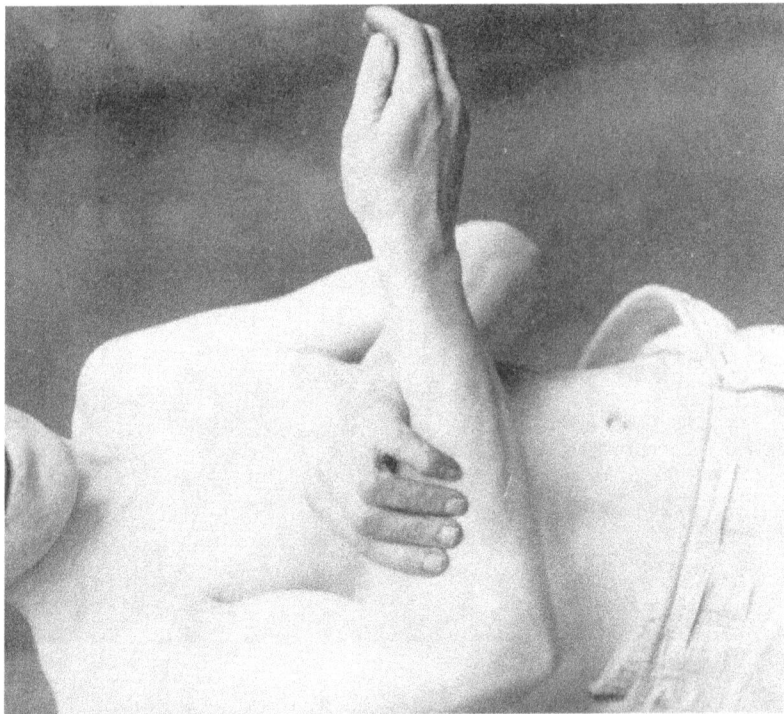

FIG 26a

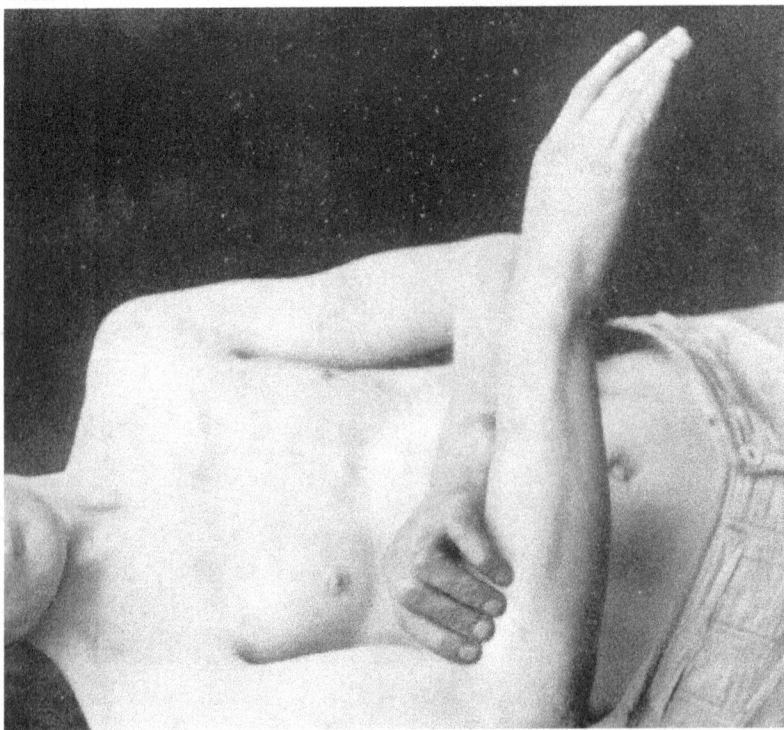

FIG 26b

Manipulation of the Exteensor Muscles of the Fore Arm. The Elbow is in Flexion. Particularly of the inner side

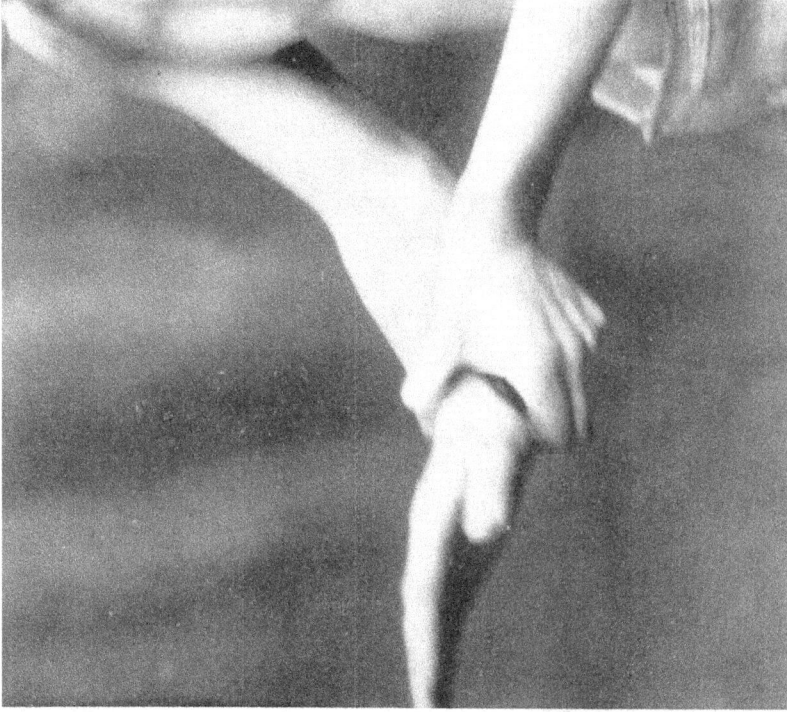

FIG 27a

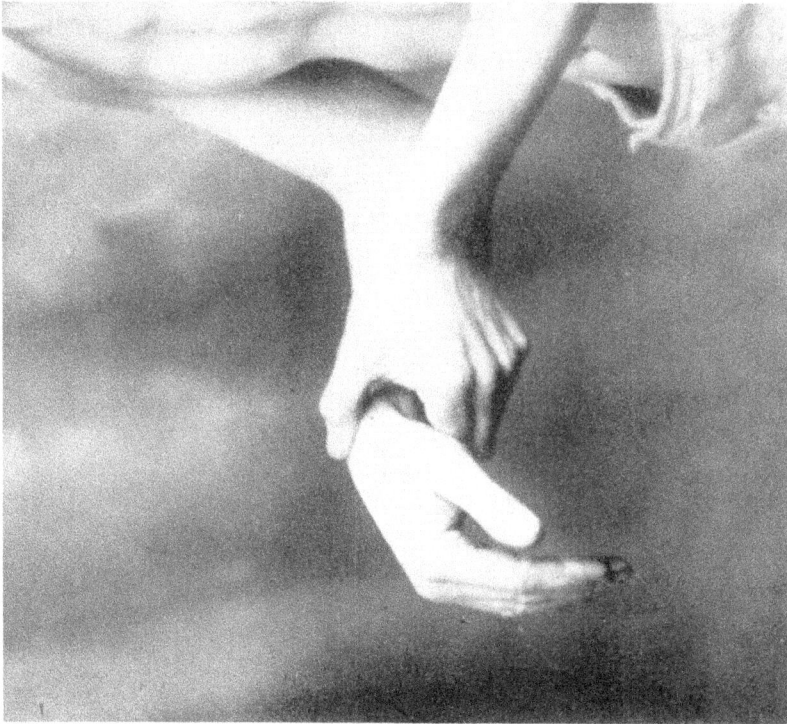

FIG 27b

Manipulation of the wrist Joint

165

Figure 28 depicts a valuable movement under which the muscles lying between the thumb and fore finger are manipulated and pressed. Like so many other places in the body, these muscles are often tender, and the tenderness interferes with the freedom with which the thumb and fore finger ought to be drawn together. Even the muscles which form the rounded musculature of the ball of the thumb in front, the opposing muscles as they are called, are sometimes found to be tender. The first and second metacarpal bones, those which carry the thumb and fore-finger respectively, are very often so, and free manipulation of all the parts, muscular, bony and articular, is advisable. It is, of course, the periosteum or connective tissue covering the bones and the perimysium or connective tissue covering the muscles rather than the bones and muscles themselves that are mainly affected, although the latter may be so also to some extent. Both hands ought to be moved or manipulated, although only one, the right, is shown in the photograph. The right is usually affected more than the left because the fact that more people are right handed than left handed leads to more stimulation and congestion of the right upper extremity than of the left. This is by no means so markedly the case with affections of the lower extremities, because, although right-handed persons are generally also right-footed, they use their legs much more equally than they do their arms.

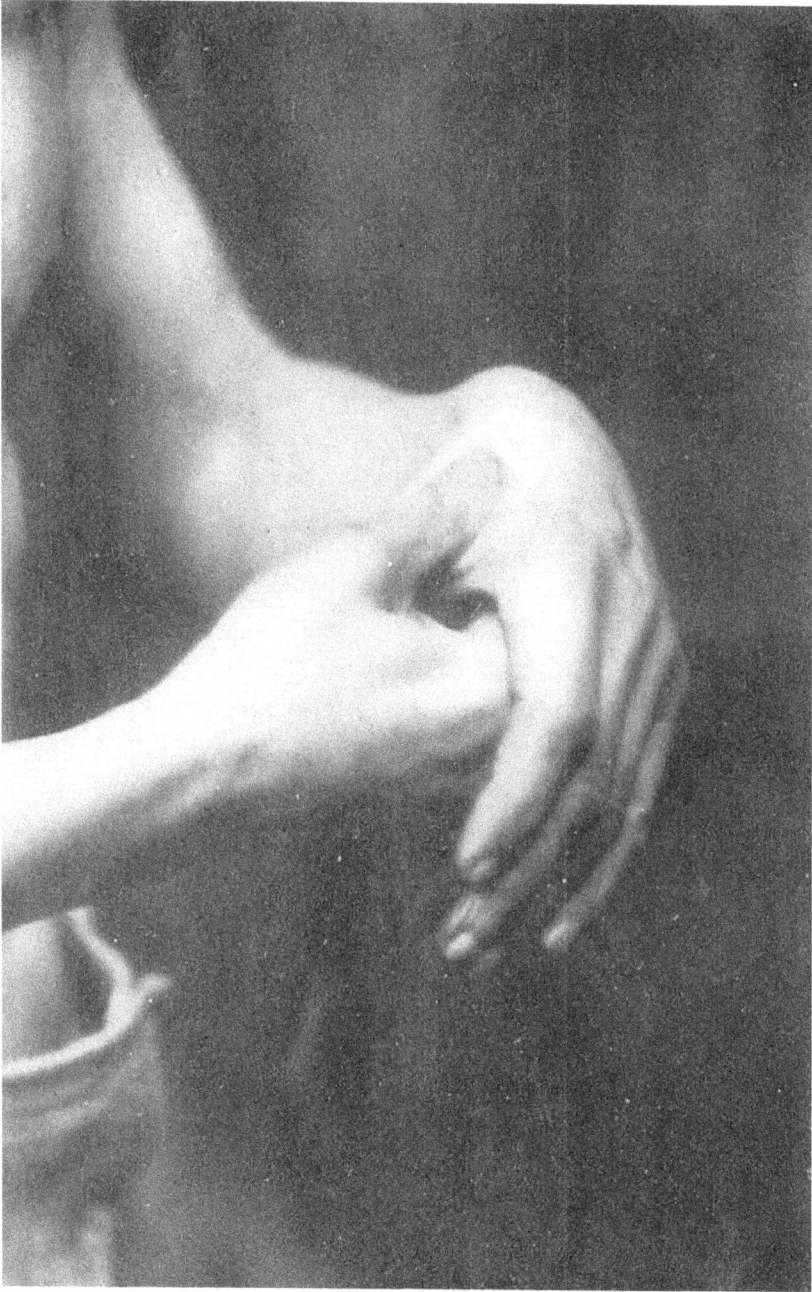

FIG 28
Manipulation of the Muscles between the Thumb and Fore-Finger

I have now described a number of the most important movements which it is advisable to perform, in order that the body may act as a fit instrument for the force of human life which procreates it and which inhabits it all through what is called life. Of course, I have not described all the pressure movements which may be beneficially instituted in the body. I hope that any person who sets into action those described will find out others whose action will be useful. No doubt this will be so. Wherever tender places are found, manipulation should be resorted to under pressure either of one's own hands or of those of a masseur or masseuse. The beneficial effects experienced induce one to go on to find out other tender places.

Those who do not believe that these tender places exist in the body will not treat them. If after what has been said anyone is sceptical as to the existence of these facts, or if he thinks that they are unproved, he must remain of the same mind. If we attach no importance to the occurrence of the infectious illnesses of early life, to the measles, the scarlatina, the typhoid and the rest that affect the children; if we see no connection between their occurrence and our mode of life, or our children's mode of life, we shall go on living as we are doing, and bear our inevitable ills as best we can. If we think that the occurrence of colds and inflammations more or less frequent, and more or less severe, of sore throats, bronchial catarrhs, stomach-aches and colics do not signify that there is something wrong in our way of living, and that we ought to alter the same if we wish to live healthier lives; if we think that the feeling of being fatigued and tired without adequate cause in work or occupation of some sort means nothing, and if we do not see the nexus or relation between this state of fatigue and congestion of the connective tissue and the subsequent or coincident occurrences of peliosis, of our influenzas, of our apoplexy, our Bright's disease, our cancer, our diabetes and our incurable diseases generally; we shall go on attributing no doubt to Fate or to necessity or to the nature of things the occurrence of evils which are of our own bringing on, and shall justify the same by uttering little proverbs about three score years and ten forming the natural duration of human life. If we really believe that the occurrence of these evils generation after generation after generation is quite inevitable and cannot be avoided, we shall make no change in our way of living so as to prevent in our successors the occurrence of the sufferings which have marked the few and evil days of our own lives. There is nothing more to be said. We who ought to use our judgment in accordance with the evidence, and to alter our conduct accordingly, will continue in the same ways that our ancestors have pursued. If we are determined to be un- convinced even if one should rise from the dead to warn us of the follies of our ways, there is no power to prevent us from coming to our determination.

The government we are under is not coercive but persuasive; and we are at perfect liberty to follow our own ways. We must use our reason in accordance with the evidence. But those of us who come to another conclusion may do differently, and we may make use of the exercises and others undescribed but which suggest themselves, as experience of the condition of the body accumulates in the surprising way it does, to win a great reward in increase of vitality and in freedom and lightness and ease of movement both of body and mind.

It seems to me from the considerations advanced that a great increase can be made to life by these means, and that the increased life will be also much more healthy and much more efficient than we are enjoying now. Of course it is not by means of the movements only that the benefits may be obtained. It is also necessary to inquire what are all the causes at work, through which stiffness and tenderness have been brought about. These, as has been said now so often, are nutritional, and bring about their effects chiefly by blocking and silting and choking the body up by the ingestion of too much food (and drink) into it. It is at this point no doubt that the chief difference of opinion, as also of practice, arises. If too much food (and drink) is the chief cause of these conditions, then plainly those who wish to recover and to remain well must eat and drink less. They must eat and drink less abundantly and they must eat and drink less often. Only a few of us are willing to put ourselves under this discipline. This kind of advice is perhaps particularly objectionable at the present time, when the love of amusement and pleasure and the undue pursuit of wealth are so dominant among our people. Perhaps; but nearly all ages in history have been characterised by inordinate love of pleasure; and the gospel of self-restraint and of self-government has never been really popular. Could we only know or understand it, wise self-restraint leads to more and greater happiness than does self—indulgence and too great love of pleasure and amusement. Neither is there any virtue in asceticism, which is as destructive in its own way as is too strong pursuit of pleasure is. In this, as in other things, it is the happy mean which is to be aimed at. And the happy mean-what is that? It is perhaps not definable to a nicety, or to a grain or two; but it is definable in general terms and even with approximate accuracy. And the true purpose of nutrition in the adult body is to restore the waste sustained by the body by the action on it of the life-force which procreates and inhabits it.

No thing can withstand the action of force without wasting and being consumed by the force. But the body has been so beautifully made, and is so carefully maintained by the force of life, that it wastes very little, probably little more than half a pound a day when doing the ordinary work of life. This is, therefore, in general terms what is required to be ingested into the body in order that it may be properly nourished and so remain fit to act as the efficient instrument of the life-force. Cornaro, as is well known, found that twelve ounces of solid food a day, and fourteen ounces of red wine was enough for him, and he lived to about ninety seven years of age on this allowance. It may, I think, be considered to be as near the mark of the average required by the body as we are likely to reach. Most of us take two or three or four or more times this amount of food; and most of us are ill in consequence of this, and die far earlier than we need do. The worst of it is that while we do live, our lives are far less efficient, as well as far less happy, than they might be. What might be done for humanity by increasing the length of healthy, happy and efficient life has been referred to in the first part of this book. It transcends human imagination to conceive, and perhaps had better be left to the imagination of each reader.

But other considerations arise, and perhaps a word may be allowable about them. It is well known that cultivation of the powers of the body and of the mind leads to the increase of them, while on the other hand failure to cultivate them causes them to remain in an infantile state, or even leads to their atrophy and decay. When we come to look at the mechanism of the connective tissue on the one hand and at that of the cerebro-spinal and sympathetic nervous system on the other, through which the various faculties are exercised, and when we think how response and conductivity and sensibility and associated sensibility and unity are all manifested through the functional action of the fibres and cells of the connective tissue, we begin to see how complicated are the facts involved and how important the structures through which they are manifested. And thus we see that these tissues form the coverings of the cerebro-spinal nervous system, through whose structures the appreciation and localisation of the faculties of response, conductivity, sensibility, associated sensibility and unity are exercised. If, therefore, we cultivate the faculties of the appreciation of these concomitant characteristics, we insensibly help to introduce, and that with a constantly increasing refinement and adaptation, the mechanism through which the higher faculties manifest themselves. A process proceeding from a cell meets a process proceeding in the connective tissue from another cell, and junction is effected so that associated sensibility is manifested. And as this mode of action is common to connective tissue and to nervous tissue, we not only find unconscious and instinctive and associated sensibility in course of manifestation, but also appreciation thereof-that is, the beginning of consciousness and of knowledge of knowledge. For if the function of some nervous cells is to act as the means of knowing, it is no doubt the function of others to act as the means of knowing that they know, and probably of others still to act as the means of knowing that we know. In other words, consciousness has gradually arisen, and even self-consciousness, we knew not how. As these faculties strengthen by use, so no doubt the mechanism through which they manifest their functions strengthens and increases and becomes better and better adapted to its ends, unconscious and conscious. It literally therefore appears that we do not know what we shall be, nor to what height humanity might attain by three or four generations of proper living. How can we know that which has not yet come into being ? But we do know that the more we aspire and reach out towards the cultivation of our own nature, and the appreciation of our place and role in the universe in which we live, the better adapted will the mechanism become to act as the means of the manifestation of the higher powers of life.

The process of development becomes like the ascent of a mountain peak which seemed to be the highest point attainable, but whose ascent, achieved, served only to show that there were not one but a whole series of new heights stretching into illimitable distance, and which were still to be scaled. Each must answer for himself what he thinks his course ought to be under the stimulus of such considerations; and perhaps the two considerations will sway him which appeal so strongly to me; first that improvement can come to us only if we aspire to it; that it is therefore dependent on our own efforts, although the effect far transcends any expectation that in our ignorance we might have formed; and second, that it is not to be through over-indulgence, but on the contrary by wise restraint, of our appetites that this improvement is to be effected. This restraint is to be not for asceticism but for efficiency. It is like the fast in the wilderness which inaugurated a unique public ministry. And if we saw the significance of the facts which in such large measure are now at our disposal, we might see that since the mouth, which is the entrance to the digestive tract, is not developed with the digestive tract, but with the face, which in turn is developed with the head and brain, which is the organ of the will, it might also appear to us that the meaning of this, or one meaning of it, may be that we must take command of what goes into the mouth. And further, as we do not lap from the dish as an animal laps, but feed our mouth with our hands, which are the organs and messengers of the will, is not this to those who wish to see and know a higher stimulus still? It is certain no doubt that the finite never will or can comprehend the infinite, but like those series in the mathematics which are always approaching infinity though they never reach it, the finite may go on continually in the effort to obtain fuller and fuller light and fuller and fuller warmth which are the symbols of the wisdom and love with which this scheme of things is conducted.

Note to page 152

1. Two ligamentous bands.

The following description is given in Quain's Anatomy 9th edition, vol. ii., p. 480. "The pericardium is fixed also in front by two ligamentous bands which pass to it from the manubrium and ensiform process of the sternum."Quain quotes Luschka as authority for this statement. These bands do not seem to have been named; but a suitable name would be the sterno-pericardial bands, as they pass to the pericardium from the inner surface of the upper and lower parts of the sternum or breast-bone respectively. They appear accordingly in the index under that name. The supreme importance of understanding their significance and their relation to *angina pectoris* is shown in the text.

END

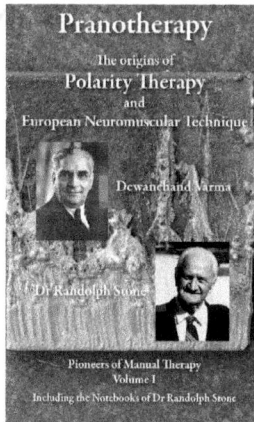

Pranotherapy

The Origins of Polarity Therapy

and

European Neuromuscular Technique

Volume 1 in the series "Pioneers in Manual Therapy"

Pranotherapy is a faithful reproduction of Dewanchand Varma's book of "The Human Machine and its Forces" which was first published in 1937. This volume also contains the previously unpublished notebooks of the founder of Polarity Therapy, Dr Randolph Stone dating from the early 1970s. Both men were pioneers of manual therapy and this volume gives a fascinating insight into the concept of healing and the restoration of health through specific hands on techniques.

ISBN 978-0956580337
Published by Masterworks International
236 pages
Profusely illustrated
www.mwipublishing.com